Retro

B A B Y

Timeless Activities to Boost Development— Without All the Gear!

2nd Edition

Anne H. Zachry, PhD, OTR/L

American Academy of Pediatrics
DEDICATED TO THE HEALTH OF ALL CHILDREN®

American Academy of Pediatrics Publishing Staff

Mary Lou White, *Chief Product and Services Officer/SVP, Membership, Marketing, and Publishing*
Mark Grimes, *Vice President, Publishing*
Holly Kaminski, *Editor, Consumer Publishing*
Jason Crase, *Senior Manager, Production and Editorial Services*
Shannan Martin, *Production Manager, Consumer Publications*
Peg Mulcahy, *Manager, Art Direction and Production*
Sara Hoerdeman, *Marketing Manager, Consumer Products*

Published by the American Academy of Pediatrics
345 Park Blvd
Itasca, IL 60143
Telephone: 630/626-6000
Facsimile: 847/434-8000
www.aap.org

The American Academy of Pediatrics is an organization of 67,000 primary care pediatricians, pediatric medical subspecialists, and pediatric surgical specialists dedicated to the health, safety, and well-being of all infants, children, adolescents, and young adults.

The information contained in this publication should not be used as a substitute for the medical care and advice of your pediatrician. There may be variations in treatment that your pediatrician may recommend based on individual facts and circumstances.

Statements and opinions expressed are those of the author and not necessarily those of the American Academy of Pediatrics.

Any websites, brand names, products, or manufacturers are mentioned for informational and identification purposes only and do not imply an endorsement by the American Academy of Pediatrics (AAP). The AAP is not responsible for the content of external resources. Information was current at the time of publication.

The publishers have made every effort to trace the copyright holders for borrowed materials. If they have inadvertently overlooked any, they will be pleased to make the necessary arrangements at the first opportunity.

This publication has been developed by the American Academy of Pediatrics. The contributors are expert authorities in the field of pediatrics. No commercial involvement of any kind has been solicited or accepted in the development of the content of this publication. Disclosures: The author reports no disclosures.

Every effort is made to keep *Retro Baby: Timeless Activities to Boost Development— Without All the Gear!* consistent with the most recent advice and information available from the American Academy of Pediatrics.

Special discounts are available for bulk purchases of this publication. Email Special Sales at nationalaccounts@aap.org for more information.

Printed in the United States of America

9-472   1 2 3 4 5 6 7 8 9 10

CB0125
ISBN: 978-1-61002-510-2
eBook: 978-1-61002-513-3
ePUB: 978-1-61002-511-9

Cover and publication design by Peg Mulcahy

Library of Congress Control Number: 2020948707

Praise for the First Edition of Retro Baby

Packed with wonderful "retro" activities and based on modern-day research, Dr Zachry shares how to avoid "baby product" hazards by sticking with the tried-and-true, fun, sensory-motor activities that babies really need. A must-read guide for the discerning parent!

Barbara A. Smith, MS, OTR/L
Author of *From Rattles to Writing: A Parent's Guide to Hand Skills*

This is a great book for any parent, but particularly for those who want to minimize the high-tech, often unnecessary, paraphernalia being pushed these days! Parents, you will appreciate the creative ideas for entertaining your baby and encouraging your baby's development.

Rachel Y. Moon, MD, FAAP
Professor of pediatrics, George Washington University School of Medicine and Health Sciences, Children's National Medical Center; editor in chief, *Sleep: What Every Parent Needs to Know;* chairperson, American Academy of Pediatrics Task Force on Sudden Infant Death Syndrome

It's great to see someone take notice of the wonderful way that experiences while awake in prone help the infant learn essential motor skills and do not require special expensive equipment. In addition, parents can be their child's first teachers of exploration, communication, social interaction, and sensory and manipulation skill using inexpensive toys. Many parents will learn that there are simple, easy ways to promote a baby's development.

Michael E. Msall, MD, FAAP, FAACPDM
Professor of pediatrics, University of Chicago Medicine Comer Children's Hospital, and cochair, Pathways.org Medical Round Table

Put down your smartphone and pick up this book. With plain-spoken, concise wisdom, Dr Zachry provides vital, research-backed information for parents of young children. Creative, interactive play with other children and adults supports healthy brain development in ways today's technology never will. *Retro Baby* provides parents fun, money-saving activities that will set their children up for lifelong success.

Mark Bertin, MD, FAAP

Developmental pediatrician, author of *The Family ADHD Solution: A Scientific Approach to Maximizing Your Child's Attention and Minimizing Parental Stress,* and editorial advisor, Common Sense Media

For my husband, Mike
With all my love

Equity, Diversity, and Inclusion Statement

The American Academy of Pediatrics is committed to principles of equity, diversity, and inclusion in its publishing program. Editorial boards, author selections, and author transitions (publication succession plans) are designed to include diverse voices that reflect society as a whole. Editor and author teams are encouraged to actively seek out diverse authors and reviewers at all stages of the editorial process. Publishing staff are committed to promoting equity, diversity, and inclusion in all aspects of publication writing, review, and production.

Contents

Foreword

Have you ever held a garage sale? I just spent a long morning watching strangers rummage through big plastic bins full of stuff I bought my 3 children (ages 8–13) over the years, most of it with the intention of helping them develop inquisitive minds and strong bodies. There's nothing like seeing all those toys spread out in my driveway to help me realize that my children didn't need the vast majority of what was out there. Even worse, some of it may have done more harm than good.

I am a sucker for marketing. When advertising executives think up their pitches and they imagine a suburban dad willing to waste money on whatever gadget will make his kids happy and offer them an edge in life, I'm the guy in their PowerPoint slides. If it sings, lights up, rolls/crawls/vibrates across the floor, or requires 12 AA batteries (not included), my kids had one. And what did they enjoy the most?

Yep, the boxes all that stuff came in (except for the batteries; they have flimsy boxes).

I didn't start out that way, no! My initial plan was to give my children only a set of alphabet blocks, 2 dolls, a truck, and a ball. But then there I was, standing in the aisle at the toy store, reading all the impressive-sounding claims on the boxes touting how the musical, flashing piece of plastic inside would guarantee my baby entry into a prestigious graduate school, and I couldn't help myself. Home it came, and after an hour or two spent untwisting the several dozen wires holding it in place, there it was, providing my offspring a full 3-and-a-half minutes of brain-stimulating pleasure before it was cast into the toy box, where it remained until it made its way to my driveway.

You, however, don't have to make the same mistake I did. You have this book. Read it. Take notes. Bring it with you to the baby store. The knowledge in this book is more valuable than shelves full of toys. With your own skills and a few household items, you'll learn how to stimulate your baby's vision, hearing, language, and motor skills and how to avoid inadvertently impairing those skills in your very efforts to foster them.

You will gain a stronger relationship with your child, and all you have to lose is dozens of bins of plastic doohickeys that, I have to tell you, bring a very low price at garage sales.

David L. Hill, MD, FAAP

Coauthor, *Co-parenting Through Separation and Divorce: Putting Your Children First*

Acknowledgments

I'd like to begin by thanking my mother, Beth Wyatt, for her love and encouragement. Thanks to my good friend Stephanie Lancaster for her support throughout the writing of this book. A special thanks to Jan Bell for being a wonderful mentor and a true friend.

Thank you to the precious *Retro Baby* models, Ava, Summer, Ellie, Virgil, and Zaiden, and to Laura Zumwalt for the amazing photography.

Thanks to my wonderful occupational therapy colleague, Barbara Smith, for taking the time to read and review this book. Susan Slaughter, your recommendations for Chapter 5 were perfect. You are an incredible occupational therapist with a gift for treating infants with head and neck issues, and I'm thrilled to be researching these important issues with you.

Thanks to the folks at Pathways.org; I am impressed by your dedication to the healthy development of children. Your informative brochures and videos on tummy time and development are valuable resources for parents as well as professionals.

Thank you to the reviewers of *Retro Baby*—Nerissa Bauer, MD, MPH, FAAP; Mark S. Dias, MD, FAANS, FAAP; Bonnie Kozial; Terri McFadden, MD, FAAP; Rachel Moon, MD, FAAP; Jennifer Takagishi, MD, FAAP; and Elizabeth Powell, MD, FAAP. Thank you also to the American Academy of Pediatrics (AAP) Committee on Fetus and Newborn; Section on Developmental and Behavioral Pediatrics; Section on Plastic Surgery; Council on Injury, Violence, and Poison Prevention; Section on Orthopaedics; and Task Force on Sudden Infant Death Syndrome. Thank you so much for your valuable feedback and input.

Thank you to Mark Grimes, Holly Kaminski, and all of the wonderful people at the AAP; I appreciate being given the opportunity to publish this book.

Finally, and most importantly, thank you to my husband Mike and our 3 children—Justin, Emily, and Hanna—for your patience, love, and support. I love you.

Introduction

New isn't always better, especially when it comes to the health and well-being of our children. Over the past several decades, tremendous advances have been made in the development of baby products and technology for infants and toddlers. These innovations, such as bouncer seats, carriers, and baby "educational" videos, are intended to make our daily lives easier and more efficient, but at what cost?

Is it possible that a baby's nervous system is not designed for the technological revolution that has taken place in our society? Can overusing baby gear, smart toys, and technology negatively affect the development of a child's cognitive, social, emotional, and motor skills? I believe it can.

I am the mother of 3, an occupational therapist, and a child development expert with more than 30 years in the field of pediatrics, and I have seen firsthand how the overuse of these "advances" can affect the development of children. In the past several decades, babies began spending more time with educational videos and high-tech toys, and the advent of baby gear brought about the trend of babies spending excessive amounts of time sedentary in plastic devices, such as bouncer seats and carriers. I've witnessed how these changes in babies' daily routines have contributed to an increase in mild developmental delays in infants, as well as an increase in the number of babies diagnosed with flat spots on their head. I've also discovered that many parents do not understand the dangers of extended equipment use and overexposure to technology.

Of course you want to give your children the best possible start in life. As a parent, you want to ensure your baby stays on track and meets those important developmental milestones. You'll do whatever it takes to help your little one build a strong foundation for future growth and development, including purchasing quality baby products that are safe and truly support learning and development.

Yet there is so much to learn. So many decisions can be overwhelming. For example, which car safety seat is safest? Do you need a changing table? How do you choose the best stroller, swing, stationary activity center, bouncer seat, and play yard? And are all of these items even necessary? The head-spinning questions never end.

You're determined to choose wisely, making sure you purchase quality items that also promote your baby's healthy development, and contemplating the countless claims made by product manufacturers is overwhelming. For example, you've heard that the toys hanging from a bouncer seat are good for babies' eye-hand coordination, while a stationary activity center strengthens their legs. Fact or fiction? Is it true that a baby walker helps your little one walk earlier? And do smart toys, baby videos, and educational programming for infants really stimulate intellectual development? I answer these questions and many more in *Retro Baby*.

This book

- Explains how crucial connections are formed between your infant's brain and muscles during the first year after birth
- Describes how the overuse of certain baby equipment can hinder child development
- Offers suggestions for daily time limits on particular pieces of baby equipment
- Explains how positioning techniques and good old-fashioned play affect your baby's growth and development in a positive way
- Includes a variety of fun, entertaining activities that enhance a child's ability to learn
- Describes how to make traditional, handmade toys to replace the budget-busting clutter on the market today

All this information helps you play a role in building a solid foundation for your child's future skills in school and life. When you use this authoritative, up-to-date source, you'll be faithfully supporting—but not rushing—your baby's mastery of developmental milestones.

What You'll Find in These Chapters

Chapter 1 explains how a baby's brain and body are developing rapidly during the first year after birth. It also describes how the overuse of many baby products can have a negative effect on development and why the nervous system of a baby is simply not designed for the techno-logical revolution that has occurred in our society.

Chapters 2 and 3 review the stages of motor skill and sensory devel-opment that occur during your child's first 2 years using clear, straight-forward language.

Chapter 4 discusses the importance of the American Academy of Pediatrics "back to sleep" recommendation. It emphasizes how to have fun incorporating tummy time into your baby's routine.

In Chapter 5, you'll find an overview of the negative consequences of overusing certain baby gear. It explains how overuse of equipment such as carriers and swings can lead to tight neck muscles and flat spots on a baby's head. On the positive side, it suggests alternative positions for fostering child development.

Chapters 6 through 10 feature specific instructions for time-tested play positions and activities geared for each developmental stage. These engaging tasks enhance your baby's strength, movement, balance, and coordination skills as well as mental and emotional development. In these chapters, you'll also find instructions for hand-making a variety of developmentally appropriate toys using common items in your home. (To write clearly and without a gender bias, I will alternate the use of "he" and "she" between chapters.)

A Starting Point

This book is all about being flexible, so I want you to keep an open mind as you read over the activities and suggestions. Certain ideas may work for you exactly as instructed, while others may offer a starting point for your own creative ideas and problem-solving. For example, if an activity involves grasping a rattle and your baby is not holding items on his own yet, have him bat at a toy rather than grasp the rattle. By meeting your baby at his developmental level, you will provide experiences that sup-port his growth and development.

As much fun as you'll be having with the activities introduced in this book, take care not to overstimulate your baby, especially in the early weeks after birth. As you play with your little one, watch for signs of fatigue such as fussiness or turning away during an activity. Then you know it's break time!

Always remember that as the parent, you intuitively know which activities suit your baby best. Trust your instincts. If your little one doesn't show interest in a particular activity, it may mean he's not developmentally ready for it. There's no rush. Simply try it again in a week or so. You will find that you naturally pick up on your baby's cues, and your sensitivity to his readiness can avoid a stressful situation for both of you.

Guidance for Your Child's Development

Throughout this book, I offer daily time-limit suggestions for using particular pieces of baby equipment. When a baby spends too much time in baby gear, it limits the opportunities he has to be physically active and explore his surroundings, and less activity is not good for baby's muscle strength and motor skill development.

Please note that the time-limit suggestions are best-case scenarios and only meant to serve as guidelines. For example, on a certain day, if a lot of travel time is necessary, reduce your baby's time in other pieces of equipment to make up for being in the car safety seat for a long period that day. If you're spending the day at the fair and your baby gets more stroller time than you prefer, he can spend more time in your arms or on the floor playing for the remainder of the evening.

These guidelines were calculated from averages to responses from more than 150 baby gear surveys completed by pediatric occupational and physical therapists. Please understand that what therapists recommend may simply not be feasible at all times in real life. Therefore, don't feel guilty if you have a busy day and your baby spends more time in baby gear than you are comfortable with. Understandably, parents have to do what they have to do to get through a hectic time. Do your best to keep the guidelines in mind, and if you get off track one day, make a point to get back on track the following day.

Avoid being drawn in by the marketing and advertising hype from baby product manufacturers. Instead, use the strategies and suggestions provided in this book to help you get "back to the basics" when caring for your little one. By limiting equipment use, being as screen-free as possible during the first 2 years, and having fun with activities included in this book, you'll guide your child's development in a healthy way.

And what's the absolute best reason to carry out the developmental activities in *Retro Baby?* They'll give you lots of opportunities to spend one-on-one time with your baby, creating a special bond that will last a lifetime!

CHAPTER 1

How the Baby Product Industry Affects Your Child's Development

More than 3 decades ago, I became a parent. Wanting to be totally prepared for my son's arrival in 1990, I had 4 major items on my must-have list: a car seat, a high chair, an infant seat, and a playpen. That's it!

How things have changed. Today, with the vast number of baby gadgets and gizmos on the market, it's easy to get caught up in the baby equipment trap. In fact, it's common for new parents to spend up to $13,000 on baby-related products during the first year alone.[1]

Without a doubt, the parenting industry has become big business. With thousands of baby products available, today's parents—especially first-time parents—have to wonder how many items are necessary. Certainly more than 4, right?

Besides wondering how many items are needed, parents can easily get overwhelmed by the vast array of choices. As a new parent, should you purchase a stroller that reclines or one that collapses with just one hand? Is a baby walker dangerous or will it help your infant walk sooner? What about the travel system with a carrier that snaps out of the car and into a stroller—how safe is that?

With my next 2 children, I got caught up in it all. By the time my youngest daughter was born, I had accumulated the following: a car seat system, a swing, a jumper, a bouncer seat, an activity mat, a high chair, a stationary activity center, a tummy-time mat, an umbrella stroller, a jogging stroller, a double jogging stroller, a play yard, a baby monitor system, and a regular double stroller. Of course, this list doesn't include the standard crib, mobile, toys, and all the equipment the grandparents purchased to have in their house for their grandchildren.

As we accumulated more equipment, not only were we spending an enormous chunk of our family budget on it, but our home also became increasingly cluttered. I can't tell you how many times I tripped over a bouncer seat or some other baby item in the middle of the night. Gradually I began to wonder, "Is all this stuff worth it? Are these conveniences meant to simplify my life actually *complicating* it?" Plus, as a parent, I felt manipulated by an industry attempting to "guilt" me into believing I needed their products. What was truly necessary?

Not only was the excess baby gear overwhelming us, but here's the kicker: I'd heard that overusing many highly touted products had the potential to *negatively* affect my baby's development. That did it! I was compelled to explore this idea further, and I was also planning to conduct research for my doctorate degree. The 2 came together beautifully. I chose to explore baby gear use as it relates to child development. Added to that was my curiosity about the effect of television (TV) and baby videos on child development. What exactly did the research say about this? I set out to discover the truth—and to tell the truth—to other concerned parents.

A Stimulating Environment

A newborn comes into this world with 100 billion neurons. What are neurons? Basically, they are the building blocks of the brain. During early life, the brain forms multiple connections among these neurons, and connections are a good thing. Why? Brain research tells us that more connections mean greater potential for learning.[2] Amazingly, approximately 1,000 trillion (sextillion) connections typically grow to connect the neurons in the brain during a child's first 3 years.[3] The number of connections that form directly relates to a child's life experiences. As parents this means you want to be sure to provide your baby with good nutrition, language exposure, and a strong emotional connection as well as touch and movement. The more balanced yet stimulating baby's environment, the more nurturing and supportive interactions provided, the greater number of neurologic connections that form.

What does this mean to parents? Whatever we do to stimulate and support our babies' development helps their brains thrive!

In addition, as new connections among neurons constantly form, there are some neurons that don't get used. So that the brain stays efficient, those unused neurons are pruned away, making room for new brain growth. This fact of nature tells us that IQ is not fixed at birth and explains why a newborn's brain doubles in size by age 3.

Naturally, as parents, we want to support this growth and development, yet we have to take a close look at many of the products on the market and carefully consider claims made about these products. For example, product advertising claims say that baby bouncers "provide hours of fun and entertainment while delighting and developing your baby's senses," and stationary activity centers "provide loads of entertainment while helping to develop walking skills." But are the manufacturers touting their goods actually telling the truth?

Retro Baby provides answers and also shows you what you can and should do to stimulate your child's brain connections with many fun, time-tested activities that don't require expensive toys and baby gear.

The Risks

By limiting screen time and baby equipment, babies have more opportunities to experience loving touch, active movement, and emotional connection. For example, when a baby is positioned in a carrier for several hours while his mother shops, he does not have the benefits of holding his head up, actively moving his arms and legs, or visually exploring his surroundings, and he experiences limited social interaction with others. Spending too much time in carriers and other baby equipment can result in what physical and occupational therapists call "container baby syndrome." This is not an actual medical syndrome. It is a term used to describe developmental problems that ensue as a result of babies being "contained" so that they don't have sufficient opportunities to move about freely and strengthen their neck, trunk, arm, and leg muscles and develop their coordination.

Let's highlight several common baby items available on the market today that are frequently overused.

Car Safety Seats, Swings, Bouncer Seats, and Stationary Activity Centers

Plastic devices such as car safety seats, bouncer seats, swings, and stationary activity centers keep a baby confined to one area; thus, if overused, they contribute to delays in developing motor skills. That's because when a baby is positioned in one of these devices, he has limited use of the muscles in his trunk, neck, arm, and legs. Instead, he's forced to sit with his hips, knees, and elbows bent. Overuse of these products can even lead to the development of flat spots on your baby's head, called *positional skull deformities* (occipital plagiocephaly; you may also hear it referred to as "flat head syndrome"). When a baby's head rests against the hard plastic surfaces of these devices for long periods, the excess pressure can lead to flattening of baby's soft skull.[4] *Please note:* It is absolutely necessary to use a car safety seat anytime your child rides in a motor vehicle, so any limits on use should only be outside the car. Also, it is best to take frequent breaks and limit travel time as much as possible in the early months after birth.

Unfortunately, the number of babies diagnosed with occipital plagiocephaly (see Chapter 5 for more details) has increased by 60% in recent years.[5] Also, research has revealed that babies who spend more time in baby gear have lower motor skill scores than those with less equipment use.[6] These devices aren't intended for extended use—30 minutes is a good time limit for most of them. Considering the risks involved, including a flat spot on the head and slowed motor skill development, it's well worth limiting baby's time in plastic gear!

Smart Toys

Smart toys incorporate computer technology that allows the toy to respond to a baby's actions in certain ways. These toys can light up, recite the ABCs, vibrate, and sing. When a little one is given a smart toy, his innate creativity and problem-solving skills aren't required because all he has to do is push a button and wait to see what happens.

When you give a baby a high-tech toy, he is typically delighted and tries it out several times. However, once he figures out what it does, the toy usually falls by the wayside. At the end of the day, he'll probably end up playing with the box the fancy toy came in more than the toy itself. A more desirable toy would promote interaction, encourage pretend play, and foster creativity. Traditional toys like building blocks and puzzles are better for your baby's brain development. Indeed, the fewer moving parts a toy has, the more creativity is required. The perfect toy engages a child's imagination while stimulating and supporting physical, mental, and social development.

Truth Be Told — Don't reach for the most costly and high-tech toy in the toy store. A toy should be developmentally appropriate and encourage problem-solving and imaginary play. For example, a simple set of building blocks provides endless entertainment and is wonderful for baby's visual and motor skill development.

Televisions and Videos

Consider the negative effects on the developmental process when a baby watches educational videos. While watching videos, he passively stares at a screen without moving or interacting with others, not to mention the overstimulation that can occur from the flashing images and sounds coming from the screen. For example, one study found that for every hour each day spent watching baby videos, babies learned 6 to 8 fewer new vocabulary words than babies who did not watch videos. So the more time babies spent watching videos, the fewer words they knew.[7]

Research also indicates that low academic achievement, limitations with attention span, obesity, aggression, and sleep impairments are associated with overuse of childhood technology.[8–12] Unfortunately, the average daily TV viewing time for children younger than 2 years in this country is 1 to 2 hours, and this time span typically increases with age.[13]

Research reveals that watching TV interferes with communication between parent and child, which in itself is detrimental to a child's language development. One study found that when a TV is on in the home, less speech is taking place; babies vocalize less and their caregivers talk to them less often.[7] On average, for every additional hour of TV viewed, there was a decrease of 770 words heard by the child from the parent. That represents a 7% decrease in words to which baby is exposed. Research has established that the number of words a baby hears directly affects his language development up to the age of 3, and the vocabulary size of a 2-year-old often predicts the language skills he'll have 10 years later.[14] Additionally, TV viewing interferes with play, and it is associated with inattentiveness and hyperactivity.

To date, limited research exists that demonstrates that learning truly takes place when a baby views commercial baby videos. In fact, several studies suggest that constant and rapid changing of scenes in videos affects a child's subsequent ability to focus on academic tasks.[15] Interestingly, a large percentage of parents who were surveyed reported letting their babies watch TV because they believed it was educational.[16] Yet when a child watches TV, his imagination and creativity are limited. Regrettably, in recent years car video players have become extremely popular with families with young kids. Many parents believe playing videos in the minivan is the perfect way to entertain their children on road trips. Although this does keep them occupied, it's likely many parents are unaware of the risks to their little ones posed by the digital screen.

Truth Be Told

In the 1970s, most all children's programming was on the weekends. Now children's programming is available 24 hours a day, 7 days a week, including channels with programming exclusively for babies and toddlers.

Electronic Tablets and Smartphones

To add to all the electronic devices available, there are interactive tablets and smartphones to consider. Many babies and toddlers absolutely love playing with touch-screen technology—and it's no wonder! The touch screen provides instant gratification with its cool images, movements, and sounds appealing to their senses. Understandably, many parents are thrilled with this interactive technology because, mostly through media ads, they've heard that babies can learn letters, numbers, words, and concepts. However, to date there is limited research studying the connection between tablets or smartphones and infant learning.

Whether traveling in the car or waiting in the pediatrician's office, it's not uncommon for parents to hand over a smartphone, laptop, or tablet to their toddler. To parents, these devices act much like a baby-sitter, and with hundreds of apps available for young children, they're increasingly appealing to little ones. Are there potential benefits or harms to babies being exposed to these interactive screens? Again, more research is needed. For older children, the interactive element allows them to learn concepts such as cause and effect and sequencing, but for babies still experiencing critical brain development, long-term effects remain unclear.

When it comes to screen time, the American Academy of Pediatrics has made a clear stance: it advises eliminating screen time for children younger than 2 years completely, linking it to language learning delays.[13] It's important to note that just like TVs, videos, and computers, tablets and cell phones have screens too.

Truth Be Told

In years past, when little ones didn't watch a video screen (including TV) as much as they do today, they played with toys they could manipulate for hours on end. They stacked blocks, tossed balls, banged on toy pianos, and played with shape sorters. This type of play develops fine motor skills and bilateral coordination (the ability to use both hands together with ease), so when children get older and start school, they can hold a pencil correctly and have the foundation needed to learn how to write.

Numerous studies have shown that children learn better from real-life experiences than screen time, especially activities that involve moving and doing.[17,18] Unfortunately, when the use of tablets, smart-phones, and computers is added to TV time, it has been estimated that the average 12-month-old is exposed to up to 2 hours of screen time a day.[16]

Truth Be Told

What are the primary reasons parents report for exposing their children younger than 2 years to electronic media? Education, entertainment, and babysitting.[16]

Although it might sound cool for a baby to learn the concepts of "up" and "down" or "stop" and "go" using technology, you can't replace the actual experience of your child physically engaging the world through play. Active exploration develops eye-hand coordination, visual perception, and fine motor skills, each of which can't be addressed in the same way on a 2-dimensional screen. It is critical for babies to learn new concepts while interacting with actual people and objects. Building, climbing, pretending, banging, stacking, and manipulating are all 3-dimensional sensory-motor experiences that can't be replicated on a screen. By carrying out the activities and suggestions outlined in this book, you are investing in your child's development and future.

CHAPTER 2

Set a Solid Foundation—Grow, Baby, Grow!

To help your little one build a strong foundation for growth and development, it's important to understand the basics of how babies advance their motor skills. This chapter reviews the stages of movement development that occur during the first year after birth.

Child development is a complex and fascinating process. Although all healthy babies have similar patterns of growth, they don't all develop at the same rate. In the past, scientists were convinced that a baby's genetic makeup directed this development. But over time, researchers have discovered how additional factors like food and shelter play a role in development. So do social factors, including parenting practices and exposure to language.

Today we know that all of these aspects work together to influence your baby's uniqueness. It's exciting to realize that as a parent, you can play a significant role in your baby's development by exposing her to colorful books, beautiful music, fun activities, and a variety of play positions.

Developing Motor Skills

Miraculously, in 1 short year (or less) your baby progresses from lying down with limited active movement to becoming upright and mobile. She will progress from sleeping 14 to 18 hours a day to engaging in ongoing exploration and from being totally reliant to becoming increasingly independent. As your infant matures, you may notice a progression in development from the head downward and the trunk outward. For example, she will gain control over her head before her trunk and legs; she'll also control her shoulders before her arms, hands, and fingers.

Think about it this way: shoulder control is necessary to be able to reach, and the ability to control one's arms is a must to use one's hands with skill. Said another way, the large muscle groups "kick in" before the small muscle groups do. Or as a physical or occupational therapist would say, gross motor control precedes fine motor control.

Truth Be Told Be careful not to overwhelm your baby with too much stimulation. Newborns need a calm and quiet environment, while 9- or 10-month-olds enjoy more liveliness. You will come to recognize your baby's signals and understand the amount of stimulation that's appropriate based on her needs.

Developmental Milestones of Growth

Although not all babies develop at the same rate, they generally follow the same sequence. And even though some may reach certain milestones later than others, it's likely the late starters will catch up to the early birds.

As you review the following developmental milestones, keep in mind that you know your baby best. If you have concerns about your baby's development, discuss them openly with your child's pediatrician.

The following examples of a baby named Noel are of typical child development that occurs over a period of 1 year. Please keep in mind that there are ranges of ages in which development can unfold and still be considered normal; however, if at any time a concern about development arises, parents should consult their child's pediatrician.

The First Month

At birth, your newborn has limited control over her body. This is because her reflexes dominate most movements. Reflexes are involuntary muscle reactions to certain types of input (see "Baby Reflexes" later

Newborn Noel

Not even an hour old, while cradled in her mother's arms, Noel opens her small, swollen eyes. Her head is still slightly pointed from passing through the birth canal, but it will round out within several days. She holds her arms and legs close to her tiny body and occasionally moves them spontaneously, just as she did in the womb. She enjoys staring at her mother's face for long periods and frequently makes small mouthing and sucking movements, smacking her tiny lips at times. Her parents are thrilled that she's arrived.

in this chapter). At rest, a full-term newborn stays in a flexed position much of the time, which means the arms and shoulders are held tightly against the body, elbows bent, hands held in fists, knees and hips flexed, and spine slightly curved inward—a position similar to the one your baby typically maintained in the womb.[20]

You may notice that when your baby is awake and on her back, she sometimes moves her arms and legs randomly and vigorously, but her little limbs always end up back close to her body. This is normal, as she is exercising and strengthening her muscles. At this point, don't expect to see much trunk or head control. Notice how when you hold her in a sitting position or over your shoulder she may try to lift her head, but she cannot maintain this effort for long. Just give her some time. She will get there!

Give your newborn plenty of opportunities to be on her tummy while awake from her first days after birth; otherwise, she may have difficulty accepting this position as she gets older. Begin by providing small amounts of tummy time throughout the day. A great way to start is to hold her tummy down on your chest while you are in a reclined position. The muscles in her neck and upper body will get stronger with every tummy-time session!

During this first month, your newborn totally depends on you as a caregiver, so hold and cuddle her as much as possible.

Baby Reflexes [19]

Name	Characteristics	Starts	Until
Asymmetrical tonic neck reflex	When lying on the back, the baby's head is rotated to one side. The arm toward which the baby is facing extends straight out from the body with the hand partially open, while the other arm flexes and the hand clenches into a fist. If you reverse the direction in which the face is turned, the position is reversed.	Birth	About 6 months
Babinski reflex	To elicit this reflex, stroke the bottom of the foot from the toe toward the heel. Baby's toes will fan out, then curl in as the foot turns in.	Birth	Around 8 to 12 months
Moro reflex (also called startle reflex)	A sudden movement or loud noise can elicit this reflex, causing baby to have a startled look and the arms to extend out to the sides with palms up and thumbs flexed. Then the arms return to the body, elbows flexed, and baby relaxes. It's often accompanied by crying.	Birth	Around 4 to 6 months
Stepping reflex	Baby makes a series of steplike motions when the sole of the foot meets a solid surface.	Birth	Diminishes around 2 months
Sucking reflex	The baby sucks when the area around the mouth or lips is stimulated.	Birth	Around 3 to 4 months
Grasp reflex	A finger or small object placed in the baby's open palm causes the hand to tighten around the finger or object.	Birth	Diminishes around 2 to 4 months; should disappear around 5 to 6 months
Rooting reflex	The baby turns the head and makes sucking motions when the side of the cheek is stroked.	Birth	About 3 to 4 months

One to 2 Months

Over the first couple of months, your little one begins to stretch out her arms and legs more frequently, and she may even surprise you as she gains a little more control over her neck, head, and trunk. This happens because her spine is becoming more flexible and her trunk, shoulder, and hip muscles are all getting stronger. These are often referred to as the core muscles, and a strong core provides a solid foundation for future motor skill development.

At this age, your infant cannot yet learn about the world by reaching out and exploring on her own, so you have to bring experiences to her. Simply take her hands and guide her in touching and exploring toys, stuffed animals, and even your face. Your baby doesn't have to wait to discover her surroundings; she has *you* as her helper and teacher!

Noel at 3 Months

Noel is 3 months old and her parents are amazed at how far she has come with her development in such a short period. While lying on her back, Dad holds Noel's favorite rattle just above her chest and shakes it. Noel stares at the rattle and with much effort swipes at it, barely making contact. "Great job, Noel! You touched your rattle," Dad says as he places the toy in Noel's tiny hand and wraps her fingers around it. He shakes the rattle as he tells Noel, "You are making noise when you shake the rattle. Shake, shake, shake!" Noel smiles broadly and brings the rattle to her mouth.

"Now it's tummy time for Noel," Dad says, rolling her over gently onto her belly. He sits in front of her. Noels lifts her head, pushes up, and supports herself on her forearms. She sees her dad sitting in front of her, smiles, and coos. "What a big girl!" Dad exclaims.

Three to 6 Months

From 3 to 6 months of age, you'll observe dramatic changes in your infant's motor skill abilities. Toward the end of the third month she'll begin to bring her hands together, swipe at toys, and touch different parts of her own body. She will also prop up on her forearms and sit upright with help. She'll need support for these activities because although her trunk muscles are stronger, they aren't strong enough to hold her body upright.

By the end of the sixth month, your baby will likely sit without support, although she may still be somewhat unstable in this position. Having a strong trunk provides a solid foundation for future balance skills, so it's good for your baby to sit upright at this point in her development. If you notice that she sits with a rounded back, she may need some support to help her stay in a nice upright position. A slumped posture may also be an indication that more time on the tummy is needed to further strengthen your infant's core.

During this time frame, baby's movements, which began as random and jerky, are becoming more controlled. You'll begin to see your little one reach for and grasp toys and other objects. At around 4 to 6 months, your baby may even roll independently from her stomach to her back. By 6 months, she'll likely be rolling from her back to her stomach.

At 4 months, place your baby on her tummy. At this point, she should be able to lift her chest off of the floor or bed when propped on her forearms. Starting at approximately 6 months of age, she'll begin to lift into a push-up position. You may even notice the beginnings of belly crawling or creeping movements, so watch for your baby to bend one of her legs at the hip and knee joint and pivot from side to side. This lets you know that her trunk and arm muscles are getting stronger. As your baby gains more control of her body, watch her engage in purposeful play. Consider play her job—for that's how she'll develop social, manipulation, and visual processing skills. During play, she'll also develop her imagination and increase her attention span. Playtime is a wonderful, healthy way to stimulate your infant's development. As you carry out the various activities in this book, be sure to keep them fun for your little one—and for you too!

Noel Is Going Strong at 8 Months

Noel is enjoying playtime with her mom. They are sitting on the floor and Noel's mother has her hand behind Noel's back, just in case she starts to topple over. Sometimes Noel uses her hands to catch herself, but not always. Noel reaches for a teething ring on the floor and grasps it with her thumb and fingers. She holds it with one hand, then moves it to her opposite hand as she babbles. Her mother watches with pride.

After several minutes of play, Noel's mom positions her daughter on her stomach. Noel still enjoys tummy time, but she doesn't stay on her belly for long. She moves into a hands-and-knees position, begins to rock back and forth, and squeals and laughs.

"You are such a big girl. I believe you are almost ready to crawl!" her mother says.

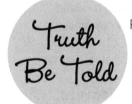

Truth Be Told

Playing with your baby provides natural occasions to practice different skills, including imitating, problem-solving, and taking turns (to name only a few).

Seven to 9 Months

By the time your baby reaches 7 months, you'll be extremely proud of her accomplishments. At this point, she is on the threshold of gaining independence in exploring the world. What an exciting time!

I remember with my children, they developed so quickly from this point forward. It's around this time your baby begins to sit up independently. If you place your little one on her back, she won't want to stay in that position for long. She has gained more control and will likely flip over onto her stomach so she can better visually and physically explore her surroundings. Once your baby can sit without support, it won't be long before she attempts to crawl on her hands and knees. With your guidance, she can learn how to rock back and forth in this position and push off to get moving.

If your baby tries to use another method of locomotion, like rolling, scooting around on her bottom, or pulling herself forward with her stomach dragging on the floor, encourage her to get on all fours in a pre-crawling position as often as possible. This sets up the important crawling stage.

Happy Birthday, Noel!

Noel's parents have to ask themselves how it can already be her first birthday? They watch their daughter as she crawls slowly across the kitchen floor, stops near a chair, and sits on her bottom. She looks around the room at the comings and goings of the birthday partyers, then immediately checks to see if Mom and Dad are still close by. She smiles when she sees them. She reaches up and grasps the seat of the chair and pulls herself up to a standing position.

"OK, it's time for birthday cake," Noel's mom says. She walks over, lifts her daughter, and places her in the nearby high chair. Noel's father brings the cake over while the guests all sing "Happy Birthday to You." After her dad blows out the candle, Noel looks at him and says, "Dada!" Everyone laughs.

Mom removes the candle and hands Noel a baby spoon, but Noels shakes her head no and drops the spoon over the edge of the high chair tray. More laughter. Noel stares at the cake. She reaches toward it, pinches off a tiny piece with her thumb and index finger, and smiles broadly.

Truth Be Told

A developing baby needs plenty of transitioning from one position to another, from side lying to sitting up to getting on her hands and knees. It's important for the trunk to rotate during these transitions because this improves baby's core strength, flexibility, and coordination.

Ten to 12 Months

During these 3 months, your baby will continue to make major progress. If she's not already crawling, it's likely she will start soon. Naturally, she'll be curious and ready to explore the environment; she'll definitely find a way to get around.

During this time, your infant will likely pull to stand, take her first steps while holding onto furniture, stand from a sitting position, and possibly take a few independent steps. Expect to see her intentionally releasing objects and picking up tiny items using the tip of her thumb and forefinger. This is called a pincer grasp.

With all this exploration going on, put safety measures into place. For example, remove all small, fragile objects from the environment; be sure to put safety locks on cabinets and drawers; cover electrical outlets and sharp edges; and place baby gates near stairs.

Crawling and Development

You've certainly been busy since your infant's birth, but as soon as your little one learns to crawl, get ready to pick up the pace even more!

Your crawling infant will have loads of fun exploring her surroundings as her sense of curiosity increases. As she gains experience crawling, she'll get stronger and more coordinated. You'll see her visual-spatial skills and self-confidence improve in the process.

Provide ample opportunities for your little one to get down on all fours and just crawl! In addition, exposing your baby to plenty of tummy time strengthens her back, neck, shoulder, and arm muscles, which makes crawling much easier. In fact, as soon as the umbilical cord falls off, you can start putting tummy time and side lying into baby's schedule during awake time. The earlier you start, the more likely she will tolerate the position. And the more tummy time your baby experiences, the easier crawling will be for her.

Truth Be Told Research has shown that babies who use walkers often exhibit slight delays with motor skills, including crawling and walking, although researchers are unsure why. Plus, baby walkers can fall from ledges or steps and injure your baby. In fact, the American Academy of Pediatrics has recommended a ban on the manufacture and sale of walkers because of the high number of injuries associated with their use.[21]

You now know that babies develop motor skills at different rates, some faster than others. Around 6 to 8 months, an infant typically gains the strength to get up on her hands and knees independently. As she experiments in this position by rocking back and forth, she gains the strength and balance needed for crawling. Before long, she transitions from rocking to moving forward on her hands and knees.

Naturally, your little one increasingly gains a sense of independence as she moves from one place to another without your help. She's experiencing a baby's form of motivation, goal setting, and goal mastery as she crawls to reach her toys and loved ones.

She also gains self-confidence as she successfully explores the environment. She even gets more familiar with not getting her way because crawling results in her hearing "No!" more often than she did as a pre-crawler.

When an infant first crawls on her hands and knees, she has a new and different perspective of the world. Crawling is good for visual-spatial skills because as she moves about the environment, she actually experiences distance, relationships, and 3-dimensional space. Crawling also provides wonderful exercise for baby's eye muscles because she has to frequently look up toward where she is headed then down at her hands when moving from one place to another.

Look out! With your baby crawling to new places, she has more opportunities to pick up, grasp, examine, and manipulate small items. This improves her fine motor skills, and strong fine motor skills give baby a solid foundation for future tasks that require eye-hand coordination, including buttoning, snapping, cutting, keyboarding, and handwriting. Just be sure nothing inappropriate ends up in her mouth! Always keep small parts or objects, balloons, toys with long strings and cords, and window treatment cords out of the reach of your baby, as these pose choking and strangulation risks. This is a good time to secure bookshelves, dressers, and other tall furniture to the wall with screws or straps. Remove all potential hazards in areas where your baby spends time.[22]

Truth Be Told

In 1992, the American Academy of Pediatrics recommended that babies sleep on their backs to decrease the risk of sudden infant death syndrome.[23] Since then, many parents have noted that their babies may start doing things such as rolling over and crawling later than other babies. However, a study showed that even though babies who sleep on their backs may reach some developmental milestones a little later, they still do them within the normal time frame.[24] So it's not anything to worry about! You need to still make sure that you are placing your baby on her back for sleep at all times (nap time and nighttime). In addition, some infants skip the crawling stage and go straight to walking. If you provide tummy time, this helps your baby to develop the necessary skills for crawling.[24] So be sure to provide your baby with plenty of tummy time, and always remember to position baby on her back for sleeping because this is the safest position.

Naturally curious about their environments, infants love to crawl and move about independently. Allow your baby to have fun while discovering unexplored territory in your home. You may notice that when she first crawls away from you, she frequently looks back to make sure you're still close. Don't fret! This is perfectly normal. The reassurance she seeks builds her confidence. Knowing you are there positively affects your little one's sense of security.

Contrary to common belief, not all babies crawl before they walk. In fact, according to a 2006 World Health Organization study, approximately 5% of babies never crawl on their hands and knees.[25] Babies who don't crawl on their hands and knees typically find another way to get from one place to another, such as rolling or belly crawling. As long as a baby is motivated to explore the environment, she'll find natural opportunities to develop basic skills such as spatial awareness, muscle strength, coordination, and self-confidence.

Why might an infant not crawl before walking? Factors such as muscle weakness, lack of interest, or limited opportunities come into play. Fortunately, parents can employ certain techniques to encourage crawling. For example, while your infant lies on her stomach, gently bend her knees, tucking them underneath her belly. Shake a colorful rattle to get her attention, then place it just out of reach in front of her. Position your forearm or the palms of your hands against her feet, providing a surface for her to push against. If she doesn't initiate any forward movement, you can gently push against her feet and give her a tiny boost.

Providing your baby with plenty of tummy time and sufficient floor space to move about also encourages crawling. Alternatively, you can sit on the floor with your legs straight out in front of you and position your baby over your thighs in a crawling stance, placing her hands and knees on the floor. Every so often, gently lift her trunk so she puts more weight through her hands and knees, and then slowly rock her forward and backward. This is a perfect exercise for strengthening her trunk and limbs. It may even provide the jump start to crawling that she needs. And don't worry if she moves backward before she goes forward when first attempting to crawl. Babies sometimes do that! Another tip is to position yourself down on her level in front of her, look her in the eyes, and use animated facial expressions to engage her and motivate her to come to you.

Note: If your infant isn't crawling by her first birthday, or if you notice she has difficulty moving one of her arms or legs, consult your child's pediatrician.

Watching your baby learn to crawl and move independently can be a truly memorable time. Take advantage of this brief period; before you know it, your little one will be pulling up, standing, and walking.

Not every infant crawls in the traditional manner. Different crawling styles include

- *Classic hands-and-knees or cross crawl.* The infant bears weight on her hands and knees, then moves one arm and the opposite knee forward at the same time.

- *Bear crawl.* It looks like the classic crawl, but the infant keeps her elbows and knees straight, walking on hands and feet like a bear.
- *Belly or commando crawl.* The infant moves her body forward while dragging her belly against the floor.
- *Bottom scooter.* The infant scoots around on her bottom using her arms to move herself forward.
- *Crab crawl.* The infant moves backward or sideways like a crab, propelling herself with her hands.
- *Rolling crawl.* The infant gets to her destination by rolling from one place to another.

As I have stressed, exploration and experiences affect a child's earliest learning, which shows why it's important for parents to encourage the development of their child's motor skills. Tummy time provides a foundation for the skill of crawling. As you now know, floor time and crawling play an important role in your child's development!

Homemade Toy Roly-poly

Your baby will love this homemade toy that encourages crawling.

Use a clean, empty, clear 2-liter plastic soda or water bottle. Squirt dishwasher liquid in the bottle, then add a bit of glitter. Fill it with water, leaving about 3 inches of space at the top. Use nontoxic glue to secure the cap in place, then shake the bottle to make bubbles. The roly-poly is ready!

During tummy time, place the roly-poly on one side of your infant just out of reach to encourage movement toward it. When your infant touches it, the toy will roll a bit. Most likely, she will move toward the toy to make it roll again.

Noel at 15 Months

Noel sits on the kitchen floor turning the pages of her favorite board book. She pats a page, looks up at her mother, who is loading the dishwasher, and says, "Mama."

"We'll read the book when Mommy finishes. Go get your ball," her mother says. Noel looks around and spots her ball across the room. She stands up and walks over to the ball, squats down, and picks it up.

"Ball!" she exclaims as she holds it up, smiling proudly.

"Way to go, Noel, you found your ball!" says her mom.

Thirteen to 18 Months

From 13 to 18 months, your child will master a number of skills. If she hasn't started walking, she will soon be walking without support, which means she is officially a toddler! As she gains experience walking, her balance and coordination improve, and before you know it she will be squatting down to pick up toys. During this time frame, she also gains greater control of her fine motor skills. She learns to feed herself with her fingers, turn the pages of a board book, and stack blocks. These new talents will make her quite proud of herself.

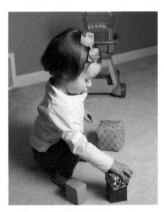

Squatting to retrieve a toy

Nineteen to 24 Months

By the time your tot reaches 2 years of age, she will likely be able to run, walk on her toes, kick a ball with one foot, walk backward, and scribble with a crayon. As her fine and gross motor skills develop, she also develops her own sense of self, which means she is discovering that she is a unique person who can think and act on her own.

Noel Is 2 Years Old

Noel is sitting in her high chair having a snack as her mom makes a birthday cake. She watches her mom stir the batter, then picks up her spoon and imitates her mother's stirring motions. Noel's mother's cell phone rings; she says, "Hello?" Noel brings the spoon to her ear and imitates her mother's greeting. She has come a long way in 2 short years!

Parental Stress and Infant Brain Development

Different experiences affect infant brain development in different ways. As we have covered, rich early experiences and lots of language exposure positively influence development. On the other end of the spectrum, negative experiences can adversely affect the development of the brain. For example, when you are stressed out, your infant can sense the stress, even during the early months after birth. When you are dealing with stress, you may not engage as readily with your baby, and your little one will pick up on your anxiety, tense facial expressions, and strained tone of voice. This can cause an increase in the stress hormones in your infant's brain, which is not good for her, especially if it happens frequently. In fact, research has found that when parents are stressed during their infants' early months after birth, their babies are at much greater risk of having behavior problems at 3 years of age.[26] The good news is that there are many different ways to relieve stress, including yoga, exercise, and laughing. The next time you are feeling overwhelmed, try this quick stress relief technique: Take a long deep breath in and hold it for 3 to 5 seconds. While you are holding your breath, tense every muscle in your body from your head to your toes. Then fully relax as you exhale.

Motor Milestone Checklists

Throughout this book, you'll find checklists to follow that will help you determine if your child's skills are developing on schedule. As you watch your child grow, you'll see how each developmental milestone builds on a previously developed skill.

Watch carefully for these events, but remember that because of the broad range of possible development within different age ranges, milestones are not set in stone. Keep in mind that every child develops at her own pace. Don't worry if your child isn't mastering these milestones according to this exact schedule. Also, when considering these checklists, be sure to adjust your child's age if she was born prematurely. For example, if your child was born at 32 weeks' gestation based on a 40-week pregnancy, you would expect her to be approximately 8 weeks behind in her development. You can stop adjusting for prematurity once your child's skills catch up to the average in her age group or by 2 years of age, whichever comes first. If you have any questions or concerns about your child's development, speak with your child's pediatrician.

CHAPTER 3

How Senses and Experiences Shape Your Baby's World

Our early life experiences shape our brains and provide a foundation for growth and development. In fact, our brains develop in direct relationship to our sensory and motor experiences. Think of the brain as a computer with its vast array of interconnections. As your baby explores his surroundings, new wires form, creating new connections.

The language he hears also leads to more elaborate wiring in the brain and enhances his learning, thinking, and creativity. His development depends on the quality of these experiences. As long as he's taking in language and sensory input, the wires in his nervous system continue to form new connections. This is why it is critical to provide a rich sensory environment with plenty of play and language during the early stages of your baby's growth and development.

When you have a feel for how your baby's nervous system works, you can nurture his development during play with the right amount of stimulation at the right time. Again, think of your child's brain as a computer composed of nerves that process information coming in from the world around him. How does he take in that information? With his 5 basic senses—vision, hearing, smell, taste, and touch—and with 3 additional sensory systems—the system that processes movement, the system that tells him where his body parts are in space, and the system that lets him know how he feels inside. As that little brain receives input from each separate system, it must be interpreted, organized, and processed efficiently so he can react appropriately.[27]

It's helpful to understand how all of these systems work. Let's address each of these senses in more detail.

Vision

This amazing sensory system exposes your child to the wonders of the world. But at birth, it's not yet fully developed. During the early weeks and months after birth important visual skills are developing, such as the ability to focus and coordinate eye movements. Eye-hand coordination and the ability to judge where items are in space also develop during this time. When your baby holds his head upright and looks around, this affects the development of visual perceptual skills (how the brain processes what is seen). Visual perception plays an important role in his future ability to read and write.

In the first days after birth, your newborn sees primarily in black, white, and shades of gray and can't focus on nearby objects. At this point, your baby's eyes aren't working together smoothly because the muscles haven't developed fully. His eyes may even cross, but don't be concerned at this early age. It won't be long before your baby will concentrate on your face and with time even discriminate colors.[28]

In their first months after birth babies prefer light and dark contrasts and distinct patterns, so keep this in mind when selecting toys and decorating the nursery for your little one. Initially, he is able to focus on objects 8 to 10 inches from his face, and by 3 to 4 months he can follow moving objects with his eyes. Around this time, he will also begin reaching for objects, which is the beginning of eye-hand coordination. By 5 months, his depth perception will improve, and he will be able to see all colors. Those sweet little eyes will continue to see better and better and by 4 years of age, your child should have 20/20 visual acuity.

Truth Be Told

Tummy time and crawling play a role in the development of your baby's near and far vision. When positioned on the stomach, he frequently has to shift from looking down at what's immediately in front of him to something across the room. This important visual skill will be used when playing ball, copying from the board to paper in school, and much more.

When your baby spends time in your arms or on his tummy, this helps refine neck and head control, thus providing a steady foundation from which the eyes work. Playtime on the tummy also gives opportunities for baby's eye muscles to develop, improving his ability to scan, focus, and use both eyes together.

As you can see, it's a building process. Neck strength is needed for head control, and head control is needed to develop visual skills. What an important time for the development of your child's visual system!

Truth Be Told

The American Optometric Association recommends talking to your baby as you walk around the room to help develop his visual system, which is related to visual-spatial integration.[29] Also provide a variety of visual input throughout the day using the activities in this book.

Visual Milestones

Here is a list of visual milestones to use as a guide in determining if your baby's visual skills are developing on schedule. Remember, these age ranges are approximate and will vary from baby to baby.

Newborn to 2 Months
- Eyes wander and sometimes cross.
- Watches adult's face when feeding.
- Prefers black, white, and patterns with contrasts.
- One or both eyes may wander out of position.
- Focuses on a toy for 1 to 2 seconds.
- Regards a toy in the line of vision 8 to 12 inches away.
- Recognizes familiar people.
- Shows awareness of hands.

Three to 5 Months
- Visually follows a toy past midline
- Follows a moving object with his eyes
- Begins to distinguish red and blue
- Develops the ability to focus

- Experiences 3-dimensional vision
- Looks at items held in his hand
- Looks at distant objects or people

Six to 8 Months
- Visual tracking skills are improving.
- Imitates gestures and expressions.
- Visually follows a dropping object.
- Smiles at self in mirror.

Nine to 12 Months
- Improves ability to shift visual attention from near to far
- Visually attends up to 10 to 12 feet away
- Develops depth perception as mobility is mastered
- Beginning to judge distances well
- Throws ball with some accuracy
- Continues to develop depth perception

Hearing/Language Development

Babies can hear sounds around the sixth month of pregnancy and the internal and external parts of the ears are fully formed by the ninth month. Remarkably, a baby knows the voices of his parents before he ever leaves the womb, and at birth, he responds to those voices by turning his head toward the source of the sound. However, the sense of hearing isn't totally intact at birth. It continues to improve over the first few months after birth, so talking to him during this time is important.[30]

In the first 3 months, your infant is easily awakened by sudden, loud noises and usually smiles at the sound of your voice. Between 3 and 6 months, he turns or looks toward a new sound. He may be easily frightened by a loud voice or noise, and he's able to repeat simple sounds.

Most new parents hate to hear their baby cry, but believe it or not, it can be good for a baby to cry. Why? Because crying in infancy lays a foundation for the act of speaking. While crying, a baby is using his vocal cords and learning to control the air flowing from his lungs.

As a form of communication, crying is how your baby lets you know if he's hungry, cold, or uncomfortable. He plays with sounds and experiments with his voice, which also helps develop the vocal cords. In the first few months after birth, your baby will make repetitive vowel sounds; between 3 and 6 months, he will start making consonant sounds. Not much later, he'll be stringing together consonant and vowel sounds, which can officially be classified as babble!

Take advantage of your little one's natural desire to communicate. Encourage your baby to imitate basic sounds such as "ooo," "ah," "pa," "ba," and "ma." When your baby begins to coo and babble, repeat the sounds he makes and use those sounds when speaking with him. For example, you can say, "Coo, oh, coo, did you say coo? You are such a good talker! You can speak so well. Mommy is so proud of how you're talking to me. What a big boy!" It's good to change the tone and pitch of your voice and to use animated voices and expressions to keep baby's attention. Also, be sure to limit the background noise, such as a loud television and music, when you are communicating with your baby so that your little one can hear you clearly.

From 6 to 12 months of age, your infant plays with his own voice, makes repetitive noises, clicks his tongue, understands simple directions, and may even imitate simple words and sounds, such as "uh-oh," "dada," and "mama." Of course, making all of these pre-speech noises requires an acute sense of hearing; therefore, it is important to have your child's hearing checked regularly and avoid ear infections.

Truth Be Told

Your child's speech and language depend on his ability to hear clearly, so always talk to your child's pediatrician if you have concerns about how your little one is hearing or how his language skills are progressing.

Language Milestones

The following checklist provides milestones to determine if your baby's language skills are generally developing on schedule. Keep in mind that there is a broad range of development possible within the different age ranges, so many of these skills will vary from one baby to the next.

Birth to 2 Months
- Smiles or gurgles to a familiar person

Three to 5 Months
- Laughs out loud when stimulated
- Smiles when you appear
- Startles on hearing loud sounds
- Makes cooing sounds
- Recognizes your voice
- Imitates facial expressions

Six to 8 Months
- Responds to name
- Shows shyness around strangers
- Babbles repetitive syllables such as "ba, ba, ba"
- Responds to changes in the tone of your voice
- Uses voice to express pleasure and displeasure
- Pays attention to music
- Puts sounds together to make 2 syllables
- Points to a desired item

Ten to 12 Months
- Responds to familiar words
- Tries to imitate words
- Says a few words such as "dada" or "mama"
- Understands simple instructions
- Understands "no"
- Is active and curious

Smell and Taste

Babies are born with the ability to taste and smell. Even though a baby's taste buds are fully developed at birth, the sense of taste continues to mature after birth and is not fully developed until approximately 24 months of age.[31] The sense of smell emerges in the fetus, and because scents cross the amniotic fluid, babies can actually smell the foods their mothers eat.

The sense of smell plays a role in a baby's ability to recognize and bond with parents and other family members. Smell and taste are involved in feeding. At birth, your baby already prefers sweet liquids and dislikes bitter or sour tastes; as he gets older, the senses of smell and taste will continue to mature. By age 8, his sense of smell will be fully developed.

The sense of smell is part of the limbic system, which plays a role in triggering emotions. So if you stimulate the limbic system through aromatherapy, you can directly affect emotions and overall alertness. This is because the limbic system is connected to the parts of the brain that control breathing, heart rate, and blood pressure. A particular scent can even elicit an emotional reaction; for example, smelling lavender can have a calming effect. Interestingly, evidence-based studies have found that babies are more interested in scented toys than unscented toys.[32]

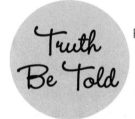

Research shows that a baby can recognize his mother's scent immediately after birth; fortunately, the natural scents of mother can be quite calming for a baby.

Touch

The sense of touch, or the tactile system, helps your baby learn about his environment and his own body awareness. Tactile input plays an important role in developing fine motor, sound articulation, and visual perception skills (the way the brain processes what we see).[33]

The skin, our largest body organ, allows us to touch and be touched, which is an important part of the developmental process. You may have heard stories of children raised in orphanages who are never touched or held early in their lives. Because these children experience limited touch, sounds, visual stimulation, and interactions, their brains are actually smaller than those of children who grow up in typical family environments. Because they are deprived of sensory input, the nervous systems of these children don't develop normally, which results in severe developmental delays and, in some cases, death.

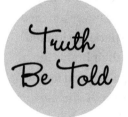

Truth Be Told

The tactile system or sense of touch is the body's largest sensory system, with several kinds of touch known, including deep pressure, light, vibration, heat, and cold.

As your baby grows and develops, he will constantly mouth and grasp his hands, feet, and even toys and blankets. Why? He wants to experience these different kinds of touch.

In fact, at birth, a newborn's sensations in the mouth are more highly developed than any other area. Not surprisingly, mouthing is one way of exploring his body and becoming attentive to a variety of sensations and textures.

As babies explore through mouthing and touching, they learn the boundaries of the body, which is the beginning of self-awareness. Babies continue to mouth and touch as a way of exploring the world well into toddlerhood and childhood.

Movement

The sense of movement, also called the vestibular system, is the sensory system that responds to moving forward and backward and rotating. The vestibular system provides us with a sense of balance because it detects motion and gravity through receptors located in the inner ear. It is through the movement system that we understand directions and realize our body position in space. This system has interconnections with many parts of the body and influences many different functions, including vision, muscle tone, postural control, balance, and eye and neck muscles. Along with the tactile system, the vestibular system is one of the first to reach maturity in early development.[34]

Truth Be Told

The vestibular (movement) system, which shows up 6 months after conception, is the first sensory system to be fully developed.

The Proprioceptive System

In addition to touch and movement, we also have a sensory system called the proprioceptive system. That's a long, fancy term meaning the awareness of one's muscle and joint position and equilibrium.

Yes, our muscles and joints have tiny sensors that let us know where our bodies are positioned in space, providing essential feedback for moving through space and maintaining balance. They allow us to feel where are bodies are positioned in space and help us explore the world through mobility. Some sensors are completely functional at birth, while others increase in function over time.[35]

But what does that actually mean? Think about it this way: The sensory receptors in your muscles, joints, tendons, and inner ear take in information about your body position and are constantly communicating with your brain, telling it where your body is located in space and how your body is moving. This system works closely with the senses of touch and movement. Indeed, if it weren't for this system, we'd have difficulty with activities that involve movement and require posture and balance.

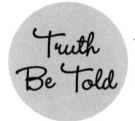

The proprioceptive system forms in utero, begins to function prenatally, and continues to develop with age.

The Interoceptive System

The interoceptive system works to regulate body temperature, emotional awareness, hunger, thirst, heart rate, the digestive system, and bowel and bladder functioning. When this system isn't functioning properly, your child could have difficulty staying alert, regulating emotions, and monitoring hunger and thirst, as well as maintaining body temperature and eventually learning toileting skills.

Because this system perceives input from many of our internal organs and constantly communicates with the central nervous system, it plays an important role in letting us know how we feel from one day to the next.[36]

Pulling It All Together: Sensory Integration

As your baby matures and continues to explore, his brain gradually becomes more efficient in coordinating input from the various sensory systems, including vision, hearing, balance, touch, and movement. The brain's ability to interpret and organize information from the senses and make appropriate reactions or responses to that information is called *sensory integration.* So if one of the senses is impaired (eg, if a baby is oversensitive or under-sensitive to touch), this can affect the process of sensory integration. These characteristics, often referred to as sensory processing symptoms, are associated with other developmental and behavioral disorders.[37]

If your baby demonstrates several of the following symptoms, discuss the issue with your child's pediatrician:

Touch

- Resists being touched and may arch when held
- Is consistently difficult to calm down once upset
- Resists tummy time
- Has problems feeding
- Has difficulty falling asleep and doesn't sleep for long periods
- Fusses during bath time and diaper changes

Vision

- Demonstrates limited eye contact
- Is sensitive to the sun and certain kinds of light

Hearing

- Gets irritable in loud settings
- Rarely babbles or doesn't make noises

Taste/Smell

- Food refusal
- Gags or vomits often with certain foods or smells

Movement

- Has delayed skills such as rolling, crawling, or cruising
- Dislikes his head being tilted backward
- Dislikes unexpected movements such as being tossed in the air or bounced
- Tends to be overly active or highly inactive
- Loses balance if he turns his head to one side to look away
- Gets fixed in postures and seems unsure of how to move
- Has low muscle tone and tires easily
- Has delayed reaching and hand skills
- Explores body parts in a limited way
- Demonstrates poor balance[38]

CHAPTER 4

Keep Your Sleeping Baby Safe and Practice Tummy Time

I often hear mothers or grandmothers say, "All my babies slept on their stomachs, and they turned out fine!" Of course I believe them, but that was before scientific research revealed that infants were 12 times more likely to be found on their stomachs than on their backs when they died of sudden infant death syndrome (SIDS).[23] If you're not familiar with the term SIDS, it refers to the unexpected death of an apparently healthy infant during sleep.

In 1992, the American Academy of Pediatrics (AAP) formally recommended that all babies be placed to sleep on their backs or sides to reduce the risk of SIDS. Later, the side position was no longer recommended because of an infant's ability to roll from the side to the stomach during sleep.[39] Fortunately, since the "back to sleep" recommendation, most babies in the United States are placed on their backs to sleep. Since the AAP recommended supine sleeping, SIDS rates have dropped significantly. In 1990, there were 130 deaths per 100,000 live infant births as compared to 35 deaths per 100,000 in 2018.[40]

Truth Be Told

Why is the American Academy of Pediatrics back to sleep recommendation so important? In 1994, the National Institute of Child Health and Human Development (NICHD) initiated a Back to Sleep marketing campaign in the United States to increase publicity about the new sleep position recommendation. The message was simple: parents, caregivers, and health care professionals were instructed to place healthy babies on their backs to sleep. The NICHD ran television commercials and public service announcements on the radio and even put display ads on buses around the country, all stressing the back to sleep message. Because of the campaign's extreme success, approximately 50% fewer infants have died of SIDS since the early 1990s.[41] It's proven to be a simple, effective way to save the lives of babies.

Reducing the Risk of Sleep-Related Problems

The back to sleep recommendation begun by the AAP is still supported by the organization. In fact, in 2011, the AAP expanded its recommendations to promote a safe sleep environment in general. The goal is to reduce the risk of *all* sleep-related baby deaths, including SIDS, suffocation, asphyxia, entrapment, and other unspecified causes of babies' deaths.

I encourage every parent and caregiver to become familiar with the following safe sleep recommendations for babies[42]:

- *Adhere to the AAP back to sleep recommendation.* Babies should be positioned on their backs for sleep until their first birthday. Avoid side sleeping because babies can roll from their side to their stomach while sleeping. Even babies with gastroesophageal reflux disease should sleep on their backs. If older babies roll into a different position, that is OK; what's important is starting them out on their backs.
- *Use a firm, flat sleep surface.* Use a safety-approved crib, bassinet, portable crib, or play yard that meets the standards of the US Consumer Product Safety Commission (CPSC). A firm mattress covered by a tightly fitting sheet is recommended, with nothing else in the crib but your baby. Do not use a surface that is inclined more than 10 degrees.
- *Your baby can be brought into your bed for feeding or comforting, but return your baby to her back in her crib when you are ready to go to sleep.* If you are drowsy or there is a chance that you might fall asleep, ensure that there are no pillows, sheets, blankets, or other items that could cover your baby's face, head, and neck or overheat your baby. If you do fall asleep, immediately move the baby to her crib as soon as you wake up.

- *Bed-sharing is not recommended for any babies.* The following situations make bed-sharing even more dangerous:
  - When your baby is younger than 4 months
  - If your baby was born prematurely or with low birth weight
  - If you or someone else in the bed is a smoker (even if you do not smoke in bed)
  - If the mother of the baby smoked during pregnancy
  - If you have taken any medicines or drugs that might make it harder for you to wake up
  - If you have consumed any alcohol
  - If you are not the baby's parent
  - If the surface is soft, such as an old mattress, memory foam, sofa, couch, waterbed, or armchair
  - If there is soft bedding, such as pillows or blankets, on the bed
- *Room share by keeping baby's sleep area in the same room where you sleep, ideally for the first 6 months.* Place your baby's crib, bassinet, portable crib, or play yard in your bedroom, close to your bed. The AAP recommends room sharing because it can decrease the risk of SIDS by as much as 50% and is much safer than bed-sharing. In addition, room sharing will make it easier for you to feed, comfort, and watch your baby.
- *Keep soft objects, loose bedding, or any objects that could increase the risk of entrapment, suffocation, or strangulation out of the baby's sleep area.* These include pillows, quilts, comforters, sheepskins, blankets, toys, and bumper pads or similar products that attach to crib slats or sides. If you are worried about your baby getting cold, you can dress your baby in layers of clothing. You can also use infant sleep clothing, such as a wearable blanket. In general, your baby should be dressed in only 1 more layer than you are wearing. Do not use weighted blankets, weighted sleepers, weighted swaddles, or other weighted objects on or near a sleeping baby.
- *Do not let your baby fall asleep on nursing pillows or pillow-like lounging pads.* Babies may roll over onto their sides or stomachs and turn their heads into the soft fabric. Or, when propped up on an incline against the pillow or lounger, their heads can fall forward, blocking their

airway. The CPSC warns that more than 2 dozen infants died between 2012 and 2018 when left on or near these products.

- *Never place your baby to sleep on a couch, sofa, or armchair.* This is an extremely dangerous place for your baby to sleep.
- *It is fine to swaddle your baby. However, make sure that your baby is always on her back when you swaddle her.* The swaddle should not be too tight or make it hard for the baby to breathe or move her hips. When your baby looks like she is trying to roll over, you should stop swaddling.
- *Try giving a pacifier at nap time and bedtime.* This helps reduce the risk of SIDS, even if the pacifier falls out after the baby is asleep. If you are breastfeeding, wait until breastfeeding is going well before offering your baby a pacifier. This means that there is good milk supply and a good latch and your baby is gaining weight well. This usually takes 2 to 3 weeks. If you are not breastfeeding your baby, you can start the pacifier whenever you like. It's OK if your baby doesn't want a pacifier. You can try offering it again later, but some babies simply don't like them. If the pacifier falls out after your baby falls asleep, you don't have to put it back in.
- *Set up a separate but proximate sleeping environment.* The risk of SIDS is reduced when a baby sleeps in the same room as a parent but in a separate crib. Place the baby's crib or bassinet near your bed (within an arm's reach).
- *Do not smoke or use any nicotine products during pregnancy or around your baby.* Secondhand smoke increases baby's risk of SIDS.
- *Avoid alcohol, marijuana, opioid, and illicit drug use during pregnancy.* The risk of SIDS increases with the mother's prenatal and postnatal exposure to these substances.
- *Don't let your baby overheat.* She should be lightly clothed for sleep, with the bedroom temperature remaining comfortable. Hats are not needed for babies when indoors.
- *Use a crib, bassinet, or play yard.* These have safety standards. Never let your baby sleep on a couch, armchair, cushion, or adult bed. Do not let your baby sleep in any sleep surface that does not meet federal standards for cribs, bassinets, and play yards. This includes inclined sleep products, hammocks, baby boxes, in-bed sleepers, baby nests

and pods, compact bassinets without a stand or legs, travel bassinets, and baby tents. (*Note:* No safety standards exist for mattresses other than crib mattresses.)

- *Avoid commercial devices marketed to reduce the risk of SIDS.* Research reveals that sleep positioners (flat or wedged mats with side bolsters) pose a risk of suffocation because a baby can get trapped and suffocate between the sleep positioner and the side of a crib or bassinet.
- *Don't let your baby share a bed.* Bed-sharing is more hazardous than when a baby sleeps on a separate sleep surface; therefore, the AAP recommends that babies not share a bed with parents or siblings during sleep.
- *Breastfeeding is recommended.* Breastfeed as much and as long as is possible. It is associated with a reduced risk of SIDS.
- *Pregnant women should receive regular prenatal care.* Babies whose mothers get regular prenatal care have a lower risk of SIDS.
- *Do not rely on home monitors as a strategy to reduce the risk of SIDS.* There is no evidence that home monitors decrease the incidence of SIDS.
- *Keep immunizations up to date.* This lowers a baby's risk of SIDS.

Keep Your Baby Safe: Avoid In-Bed Sleepers/Beside Sleepers

Many mothers use co-sleepers, also called bedside sleepers, so their babies can conveniently sleep close to them for nursing. To date, the US Consumer Product Safety Commission has not established safety regulations for these products,[43] and the American Academy of Pediatrics (AAP) does not recommend co-sleeping. There is a risk of the baby suffocating, and a sleeping parent may roll over onto a sleeping baby, resulting in the child's death. If one parent weighs more than the other, the in-bed sleeper will tilt toward that parent and the baby could roll into the side. A separate crib, bassinet, or portable play yard with fixed sides is recommended by the AAP.

- *Review these safe sleep practices with everyone who cares for your baby.*
  This includes child care staff, babysitters, grandparents, and friends.
  Make sure every individual who cares for your baby is aware of safe
  sleep practices.

Increase in Flat Spots Reported

Thanks to the Back to Sleep campaign, thousands of babies' lives have
been saved. Interestingly, several years after the back to sleep recommendation, pediatricians and therapists began noticing a sudden rise
in babies diagnosed with flat spots on their heads. They also noticed
an increase in the number of infants with mild delays in gross motor
skills, such as rolling over and pulling up.[44] Why? Before the back to
sleep recommendation, babies spent most of their days playing tummy
down on a blanket spread out on the floor, but that changed. After the
recommendation, it seemed that parents were not putting their babies
on their stomachs for play because of a fear of SIDS.[45] For that reason,
in 1996 the AAP stepped in and formally recommended that parents
provide babies with supervised playtime on their stomach. Providing
tummy time would not only promote growth and development but
would prevent flat spots from forming on a baby's head.

Unfortunately, mild motor delays and misshapen heads are still on
the rise, even after the AAP tummy-time recommendation.[46]

In 2017, several colleagues and I conducted a study that revealed that
parents of infants diagnosed with cranial asymmetry reported that their
infants received much less tummy time than those without a diagnosis
of cranial asymmetry.[47]

Why do parents fail to give their babies this much-needed tummy
time for play in such large numbers? It's possible that with the emphasis
on back to sleep, many parents are still misinterpreting the AAP recommendation and are fearful that SIDS might occur while their babies
are awake and positioned on their tummies. Although the back to sleep
message has been well conveyed, the critical need for tummy time
needs to be communicated to parents and caregivers.[48]

As a pediatric occupational therapist, I'm constantly being asked,
"What's the big deal about tummy time?" I always explain how tummy
time is important in many ways. It plays a role in organizing a baby's

Tummy-Time Woes

Laura lifted her daughter Mattie out of the carrier and cradled her infant in her arms. They had just returned from the pediatrician's office where Mattie's 2-month well-baby checkup had gone wonderfully. Mattie had gained 1 pound 12 ounces and grown 1½ inches in only 1 month!

As far as Laura was concerned, the only troubling conversation she'd had with her pediatrician addressed the topic of tummy time. The doctor had reminded Laura how Mattie should be spending at least 15 minutes 3 to 4 times daily on her stomach during supervised playtime. Laura had told him how Mattie hated being on her stomach and wailed in protest when they tried tummy time. The pediatrician assured Laura that Mattie would get used to being on her stomach. He instructed her to start out gradually and build up to the 15-minute, 4-times-a-day goal.

"Oh well, here we go," Laura said as she placed Mattie on the bed, carefully positioning her on her stomach. Laura grabbed a nearby rattle and shook it to get Mattie's attention. Her daughter turned her head to one side for several seconds, then put her head down and nuzzled her nose into the bedspread. After turning her head in the other direction, she began to whimper, and within minutes, the whimpers had turned into full-blown screams.

"Forget this," Laura mumbled. She scooped up the crying baby and soothed her. "I can't just let her scream and cry. Tummy time just isn't worth it."

Can you relate to Laura's experience?

nervous system and develops the muscles in baby's neck, shoulders, arms, and trunk. These muscles play a critical role in the foundational motor skills of rolling over, pulling up, and sitting up.

Unfortunately, many parents still aren't aware of the importance of tummy time, and many babies don't tolerate the tummy-time position. In one research study I conducted, I surveyed the parents and caregivers of babies in the waiting rooms of 4 pediatric clinics. I asked if they were aware of the AAP tummy-time recommendations and the potential complications from limited tummy time. I also asked how much daily tummy time their babies were receiving. (The AAP recommends that tummy time begin on baby's first day home from the hospital to be carried out 2 to 3 times daily for 3 to 5 minutes per session, with the amount of time to be gradually increased as baby increases tolerance for the position. The AAP suggests that tummy time take place after diaper changes and naps,[49] which equates to approximately 40 to 60 minutes a day.)

The results of my study shocked me. I learned that 25% of the caregivers studied had no awareness of the AAP tummy-time recommendations, nor did they understand the complications of babies not having daily tummy time. Of those aware of the importance of tummy time, 35% reported their babies would not tolerate being placed on their stomach for play. So even when these parents and caregivers knew the potential complications, when their babies fussed or cried, they cut back on tummy time—to 15 minutes or less each day![50] Parents consistently shared that their babies would fuss and cry with every attempt, saying things like, "My baby absolutely hates it; she just won't tolerate tummy time, and she screams every time I try!" I could hear the frustration in their voices.

Keep Your Baby Safe: Avoid Drop-side Cribs

In 2011, the US Consumer Product Safety Commission banned all cribs that have one moveable side that drops down. There have been instances in which the drop side disengages from its hardware and becomes detached, forming a gap where the baby can become entrapped and suffocate. This can happen even in the absence of up-and-down movement of the drop side. Unfortunately, more than 30 baby deaths have been caused by these cribs since 2000. It is best to purchase a crib that was manufactured after June 2011. *Note:* If your crib is older than 10 years, you should replace it—it is not up to current safety standards.[51]

Because I often work with babies who resist being positioned on their stomach, I'm highly familiar with this frustration. But I know that with time and a few simple, effective techniques, any baby can adjust to tummy time. There are ways to introduce tummy time and increase tolerance without making parents' and baby's life miserable. In fact, the result can be the total opposite of miserable because tummy time provides opportunities to spend one-on-one time playing with your baby!

Tummy Time and Side Lying

If your baby doesn't tolerate tummy time—and even if she does— I encourage you to try the following activities:

Activity #1: Tummy to Tummy

It's a good idea to begin exposing your baby to tummy time while you're both still in the hospital. The earlier you start, the more likely your baby will accept the stomach as a natural position. In fact, before the umbilical cord has fallen off, you can position your newborn on your stomach or chest while you are awake and in a reclined position on a chair, bed, or floor (with a pillow to support your head), tummy to tummy with baby. Take this perfect opportunity to socialize with your newborn and encourage lots of eye contact. Talk in animated tones and use exaggerated expressions to get her to look at you. It's a special time to bond tummy to tummy.

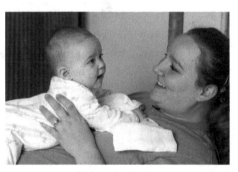

Tummy to tummy

Truth Be Told

Placing your baby on her stomach provides a nice stretch for the muscles throughout her neck, jaw, and mouth. Think about how she has to stretch her neck to look up and around during tummy time— great for muscles used during future speech and language skills. Encourage this stretch by holding a colorful toy or rattle just above her eye level so she'll have to raise her chin to see it.

Activity #2: Lap Time

You can also position your baby tummy down across your lap lengthwise while providing head support. Remember to keep her head aligned with her body. If she falls asleep in that position, just transfer her to the bed (but place her down to sleep on her back). For more stimulation, slowly raise and lower your legs at the same time, then move them slowly from side to side. This motion will likely calm your little one.

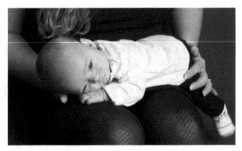

Lap time

Babies need to be exposed to a variety of textures throughout the day, and tummy time is the perfect opportunity to accomplish this. When your baby is on her tummy, the skin on her stomach, legs, arms, and face touches the surface on which she is lying. The most natural place to play is on a clean floor, a nap mat, or blankets of different textures. (*Note:* Blankets should be secured so they don't slide around when baby moves her arms or legs.) As she moves her body, arms, and legs against the surface, the friction that is created lets her know where her body is located in space. Additionally, your baby will gain strength and flexibility during tummy time. Dressing your little one in an infant body suit (eg, onesie) for tummy time allows her to feel the various textures on her arms and legs. Better yet, if the room is warm enough, just dress her in a diaper!

In her informative book *Building Babies Better,* physical therapist Roxanne Small recommends placing baby on a slick surface such as clean, vinyl flooring. The smooth surface provides a positive sensory experience, and because there's less friction than on other kinds of flooring, it requires less effort for baby to move her arms and legs. As a result, your baby is more likely to enjoy the position. For a totally different sensory experience, Small suggests stripping your baby down to her diaper and applying a small amount of grape-seed oil to the trunk, arms, and legs.[52] (*Note:* Only apply oil or lotion that you have previously used with your baby, or check with your child's pediatrician beforehand about how to test for allergies to these substances.)

Tummy time also allows your baby to visually explore the environment in a new way. When positioned on her back, she can see only the ceiling and whatever is directly around her. But on her stomach, she uses her muscles to lift her head and see the world at eye level, giving her a completely different view of the world—a new perspective!

Truth Be Told

Babies first experience texture, size, shape, shade, and color through visual exploration, so it's a good idea to occasionally provide visual stimulation for your baby. Appropriate visual stimulation helps with the development of vision, and having strong vision early in life promotes attentiveness and encourages curiosity.

An important reminder: once your baby starts participating in tummy time, be sure to provide supervision. In this world of distractions, your phone will ring or you'll get called to another room, but stay with your baby because the AAP recommends that tummy time be supervised. If your baby was born premature or has reflux disease or special needs, speak with your child's pediatrician about tummy time. Some babies need special consideration.

Keep Your Baby Safe: Avoid Inclined Sleepers

Inclined sleepers position baby on an incline, which can cause the baby's chin to drop toward the chest and block the airway, possibly resulting in suffocation. The US Consumer Product Safety Commission reports that there have been at least 73 infants deaths related to infant inclined sleep products.[43]

Activity #3: Side Lying With Support

Side lying is a great alternative to tummy time if your baby doesn't tolerate being on her stomach. Place your baby on a blanket on her side; if needed, prop her back against a rolled-up towel for support. If her head needs support, place a small, folded washcloth under her head. Both of baby's arms should be in front of her, and you should bring her legs forward at the hips and bend her knees to make her comfortable. Don't forget to distract your baby with a fun toy or read her an entertaining book while she's in this position.

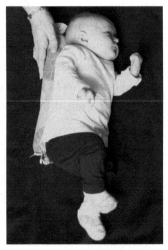

Side lying. Always provide supervision when using a bolster for positioning.

It is best to set up a regular time for tummy time and side lying, such as after naps, baths, or diaper changes. Just be sure to have a plan in place and take care to vary your baby's position every 10 to 15 minutes during playtime.

Strive to expose your baby to a variety of positions throughout the day, including time spent in your arms and on your lap. Remember, babies crave emotional interaction and connection with their parents. It's my hope that tummy time and side lying prove to be rich, rewarding experiences for you and your baby.

Truth Be Told

Be on the lookout to find something your baby likes—a song, a favorite rattle—and go with it! When necessary, use distraction techniques to entertain your baby while she's in these positions. Many simple products exist to engage babies, including baby-safe mirrors and developmental toys that nest and stack. Select basic toys that your baby loves and only bring one out at a time during tummy time and side lying; better yet, provide your baby with the handmade toys included in this book.

You'll see that when these items of interest are nearby, your baby will be more likely to lean, shift weight, and reach for them—exactly what you want! Bearing weight and reaching strengthens the muscles needed to allow baby to push up against the floor and stretch out her elbows. This is one more step in the developmental process toward crawling.

Tummy-Time Resistance

If you have waited until your baby is older than 1 month to try tummy time, it's likely that she will cry when you put her in this position. Many infants dislike tummy time because they simply aren't used to being stomach down. Your baby's neck, shoulder, and back muscles are probably weak, which makes it difficult for her to lift and hold her head upright. If she has loose or tight muscles or joints, tummy time can be especially difficult.

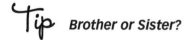 **Brother or Sister?**

Does your baby have siblings? Suggest they play nearby when your baby is having tummy time. This may provide just enough distraction to extend the amount of time your baby spends on her tummy. Tell her brother and sister to act silly or sing a song for entertainment.

Because of these factors, your infant may protest by crying or refusing to lift her head. Never force an infant to participate in tummy time if she's extremely fretful and upset. Rather, introduce the position when she's rested, well fed, and in good spirits with a fresh diaper. Start with 30 to 45 seconds once or twice every hour, then gradually increase the length of each tummy-time session. Be sure to include plenty of side-lying time as well, as this position takes pressure off of the back of your baby's head.

By listening carefully to your baby's protests and watching her body language, you'll know when the time is right to increase the length of her tummy-time sessions. Remember, your infant may initially grunt or make funny noises because tummy time is hard work. Listen carefully to determine whether she's working to maintain the position or actually uncomfortable.

Begin small and work your way up. By introducing tummy time gradually, babies usually learn to tolerate this position within a short period.

Find an activity your baby likes and go with it! If she resists tummy time, use a favorite rattle or song to distract your baby every second

Tip *Tummy-Time Toolbox*

Create a "tummy-time toolbox" of toys for baby. Take a small basket or bag and fill it with your baby's favorite toys so you can easily grab them at a moment's notice. Make sure it's portable so you can take it with you if you're headed out of the house. Don't overfill it, and when you notice your baby is starting to get bored with what the bag includes, alternate the toys. You want to keep your baby stimulated and interested, as novelty is always fun for baby!

she's in the position. By providing frequent breaks, gradually increasing time spent on the tummy, and using the various recommended techniques, your infant's tolerance will improve. Keep all of the benefits in mind. With consistent tummy time, your baby's neck, back, and arm muscles will continue to get stronger. Once again, be sure to keep your baby occupied with colorful toys to play with.

Be aware that some babies may resist tummy time because of stomach issues such as reflux, and tummy time may actually help a baby with this condition. If your baby has reflux, be sure to consult with your child's pediatrician.

The keys to helping a baby who's resistant to tummy time are to start gradually and distract, distract, distract. Understand that this position is challenging for infants, especially those who haven't been exposed to it consistently from an early age. Apply the suggested techniques for slipping tummy time into your baby's regular routine and try your best not to get discouraged. Your baby may sense your discouragement, which will only make the situation more stressful for both of you. Yes, a fretful, crying baby is upsetting, but don't give up at the first whimper. Sing, make a silly face, or pull out one of your baby's favorite toys as a distraction. Remember, tummy time gives you the opportunity to bond with your baby in a special way.

It's important to keep in mind that it's also good for your baby to spend time playing while positioned on her back. This is a nice alternative when baby has had enough of tummy time. While positioned on

Have a Tummy-Time Routine

Make a routine out of tummy time by rolling your baby over on her belly after every diaper change or just before bedtime. Having a schedule makes it easier to remember tummy time, and your baby will likely come to anticipate the routine.

her back, baby has the opportunity to explore her hands and feet, which plays a role in the development of eye-hand and eye-foot coordination and helps with body awareness in general.

You'll likely become more enthusiastic about tummy time as you see your little one gaining skills. So enjoy your time together, and odds are your little one will feed off your enthusiasm!

CHAPTER 5

Prevent Positional Skull Deformities

The Martins' daughter, Lizzie, was born prematurely, which placed her at risk for developing flat spots on her head—preemies' skulls are softer than those of full-term newborns, and they often don't have the neck strength to reposition their head independently.

In this case, Lizzie had a slight flat spot that began in utero, something that happens frequently due to baby's head resting on mother's pelvis. At birth, it was evident Lizzie had flattening on the right side of her head. A fussy baby, she didn't like to be held or comforted. Jennifer, Lizzie's mother, found that one of the few things that would calm Lizzie down was spending time in the swing. Best of all, the swinging motion helped her fall asleep! And once asleep, Jennifer didn't chance waking her up, so she usually let Lizzie finish her nap in the swing.

Unfortunately, because Lizzie was on an incline while in the swing and as a young baby had little trunk control, her trunk slumped, and her sleeping head naturally rested on the flat spot that had already formed prior to her birth.

Have you ever been at the supermarket in the line behind a parent holding a baby and noticed a large flat spot on the back or side of the baby's head? It's likely you have; this condition occurs more frequently due to factors like back sleeping, limited tummy time, and the overuse of baby gear.

Before many babies are even born, parents tend to invest in an expensive assortment of baby supplies including baby gear, bedding, and toys. Of course it's good practice to have the necessities before your baby arrives, but you now know why it is a good idea to take a close look at what's truly necessary.

Although the baby equipment surge encroaching on our society offers convenience, it's not necessarily good. The baby product industry wants parents to believe that having a baby means spending enormous amounts of money on expensive furniture, clothing, and gear to ensure your baby is safe, trendy, and smart. But does your baby really need all of that stuff?

Many babies spend long hours in equipment such as bouncy seats, swings, and carriers, but as I have stressed, the overuse of these products in the home can have a negative effect on a child's sensory and motor skill development. Because detachable car safety seats for babies can double as infant carriers, this can be even more problematic. Has your baby ever fallen asleep in the car seat while you were running errands, and when you got home, you took the carrier into the house and left baby in it to nap because you didn't want to wake him? If you said yes, please don't do this again!

First and foremost, by doing this, in effect you're teaching your baby to be a light sleeper. It's best if babies learn to fall back asleep when they're moved from one location to another while asleep. Of course, it's much easier on you to leave your baby sleeping soundly in the carrier when you have lots to do. However, when your baby's head rests in the same position for too long against the surface of a carrier, swing, or stroller, the pressure can result in a flat spot. Don't forget how soft and flexible your baby's head is at this young age. In addition, according to Susan Klemm, MS, OTR/L, the flexed position encouraged by the carrier is not good for baby's motor skill development, and the incline of the carrier can cause him to slump because it provides limited head and trunk support (personal communication, March 2021). Most importantly, remember that the American Academy of Pediatrics recommends that babies sleep on a firm, flat surface. Save car seat time for traveling, when the seat and straps protect your child in case of a collision.

Baby Gear Use and Development

Interestingly, research has even revealed a relationship between baby gear use and children's scores on developmental scales.[53] That means

$\mathcal{T}$ip   **No Sitting Around in Plastic Equipment at Child Care, Please**

If your child attends child care, make sure the classroom teachers know that he should sleep on his back and play on his stomach. This includes limiting time spent on his back on a nursing pillow and being under the activity mat on his back. Instead of perching him in baby gear throughout the day, tell them you prefer that he spend plenty of time playing on his tummy.

babies who spend more time in equipment than the test group score lower on motor skill scales than those who spent less time in gear.

Obviously, no parents want their child's development hindered by the overuse of baby gear. If you think about the risks involved—especially a flattened head and reduced motor skill development—these issues alone should convince you to limit your baby's time in plastic! I recommend no more than 15 to 30 minutes at a time in a bouncer seat, swing, or similar equipment. Don't let your baby spend more than 2 to 3 hours a day (total) in plastic equipment, and remember, less is better. (If you're traveling or have a long drive to work, find a way to adjust the schedule each day to make up for the continuous hours of sitting.) Most importantly, always use car safety seats when traveling with your baby in a moving vehicle.

Positional Skull Deformities and Torticollis

The medical term for positional skull deformities is *occipital plagiocephaly*. The word plagiocephaly literally means "oblique head." When viewed from above, the head has a parallelogram appearance caused by constant pressure to the back of one side of baby's head.[54] Occipital plagiocephaly usually results from prolonged pressure on the back of the head, causing it to flatten unevenly across the back, thus resulting in an altered head shape. The height of the back of the head may also be high.[55]

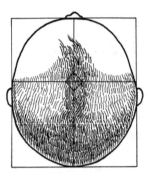 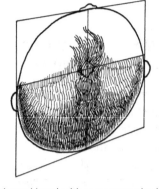

Evenly shaped head   Misshaped head with one ear pushed forward

These conditions occur because a baby's skull bone, as noted earlier, is extremely soft and flexible. The soft skull allows for the impressive brain growth that occurs during a baby's first year after birth. Yet when a baby stays in one position for too long, pressure prevents the skull from developing a normal shape. However, some babies show a preference for sleeping or sitting with their head turned in one direction most of the time. For some babies, this is because of tightness of the muscles on one side of the neck (see the Positioning Tips section later in this chapter).[56] When the head is constantly turned to one side or stays in the center, the consistent pressure molds the skull so that a section is flattened instead of rounded. This can occur quickly within the first 2 months or more gradually over 3 to 6 months. Additional factors that have been associated with positional skull deformities are being firstborn, prematurity, limited exposure to tummy time, and not altering baby's head position during sleep. While most babies who have positional skull deformities develop normally, some research has suggested an association between positional skull deformities and neurodevelopmental delays. However, none of the studies have shown that these skull deformities cause the neurodevelopmental delays.[57,58]

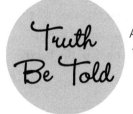

About 85% of babies diagnosed with torticollis or tight neck muscles also have plagiocephaly.[59]

If a baby experiences intrauterine constraint, he may be born with torticollis. In this condition, the neck muscles shorten on one side, causing baby's neck to turn in a twisted position, tilting his head to one side with his chin often pointing to the other side. It contributes to positional skull deformities because the baby's head tends to always be turned in the same direction, thus causing pressure against the same side.[60] Torticollis can be treated with stretching exercises with a physical or occupational therapist, who will also usually provide parents with exercises to do at home.[61] If you suspect your baby has torticollis, consult with your child's pediatrician immediately. By the same token, if your baby only sleeps with his head in one position (eg, just tilted to the left) he is at risk for plagiocephaly, which can lead to future problems with fitting into safety helmets for sports or work. If you see your baby doing this, please discuss it with your child's pediatrician.

Positioning Tips

Activity #1: Together Time

Stay in close physical contact with your baby as frequently as possible. Soft front carriers are perfect for this because baby can actually feel the parent's heartbeat, and the movement is good for baby's sensory system. These carriers provide a familiar, comfortable sensation and remind baby of being in the womb, yet baby still has to use his muscles, and he receives sensory feedback while in the carrier. Interestingly, research suggests that carrying baby in this way even promotes attachment.[62] When baby gets older, there are carriers that attach to your back, which is good for your infant's head control and visual development. They provide the opportunity for an infant to hold up his head and look around as mom or dad moves about the environment. Another plus is that these carriers free up your hands, so you can go about your daily routine while baby is right there with you. Just be sure not to overdo it. If you notice any back pain or fatigue, that means it's time to take a break. Also be cognizant of how your baby is resting his head against you; if he has a preference, be sure to reposition him frequently to the other side.

Keep Your Baby Safe: Soft Baby Slings

In recent years, there have been a number of baby deaths and injuries associated with the use of soft baby slings. Babies have fallen out of slings, and babies with limited head control (younger than 4 months) are at risk of suffocation. Take care when babywearing by reading product information carefully and selecting a front or back carrier that is appropriate for your baby's developmental level. When using a sling, be sure that your baby is positioned upright and his nose and mouth are not obstructed by anything. Avoid products that curl your baby into a C shape, as this can block your baby's airway. If you need to bend down when wearing the sling, remember to bend your knees while keeping your upper body straight. And don't wear your baby sling when you are cooking. If you breastfeed your baby while he is in the sling, make sure to position him upright after breastfeeding is finished.

Activity #2: Changing Head Position

If you bottle-feed your baby, make a point to rest his head on your left arm for a while, and then switch to your right arm. A simple way to remember this is to adjust baby's position after each burp. When spoon-feeding baby in a high chair, occasionally alternate the side on which you sit. Also, don't forget to alternate the hip or arm with which you carry your little one. I always found this especially challenging because I'm right-handed, so to keep my right hand free, I found that my first instinct was to hold my children on my left side. It took extra effort to remember to alternate sides!

Altering your baby's environment by changing the position of interesting items like toys and mirrors in the crib and stroller will encourage your baby to change his head position as well.

Activity #3: Alternate Sleeping Positions

Frequently alternate the way you place your baby to sleep. One night, have him sleep with his head toward one end of the crib. The next night, have him sleep with his head toward the other end of the crib. Because babies often look toward a particular direction (where the light in the hall is, for instance), alternating baby's body position nightly will help keep your baby's neck flexible.

Truth Be Told

If a flat spot is identified before 3 months of age, repositioning (changing the baby's body orientation in the crib, carrying the baby, or offering more tummy time) can be successful in stopping the progression of plagiocephaly and even reverse the flattening.

Preventing Positional Skull Deformities

Thankfully, occipital plagiocephaly does not affect brain growth or cause developmental delays in most cases. In extreme plagiocephaly cases, a baby may have an ear shifted slightly forward of the opposite ear, and the ear or cheek may protrude. In rare and extreme cases, severe untreated plagiocephaly may contribute to psychosocial issues related to appearance.[63]

Occasionally evaluate your baby's head shape by viewing his head from various angles, including the sides, back, front, and top. In fact, looking at your baby's head from the top down is the best way to notice the beginnings of plagiocephaly.

Since the back to sleep recommendation in 1994, the number of plagiocephaly cases has increased by 50% to 60%, and the number of torticollis cases has also increased significantly. Fortunately, these conditions can be corrected with position changes (ie, the baby's head is at one end of the crib one night but at the other end of the crib the other night so he has to turn a different way to look toward the bedroom door) in conjunction with occupational or physical therapy.[64]

More importantly, they can be prevented by stretching your baby's neck muscles, making regular position changes, and limiting your baby's time in baby gear. And don't forget tummy time and side lying while baby is awake and being observed by you or some other responsible adult! Be sure to start these practices soon after birth and work up to at least 15 to 30 minutes per day by the time your baby is 2 months old.

Follow through with these suggestions to keep your baby's neck flexible and reduce the risk of a flat spot forming.

Activity #1: Musical Chairs

When your infant starts sitting in a high chair, occasionally rotate the chair to different spots around the table throughout the week. Move where your baby plays to different parts of the room. Why? If your baby is put in the same spot of the room all the time, he'll tend to turn or tilt his head in the same direction to see the central activity. Constant change allows him to turn his head and stretch his neck in different directions to see what's going on.

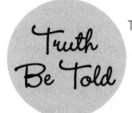

Torticollis is frequently present at birth. Physicians believe that tightness in the neck muscles may be caused by trauma at birth or because the baby is in an abnormal position while growing in the womb.

Activity #2: From One Side to Another

Approach and talk to your baby from different sides. Also, vary how you hold your baby. For example, hold him upright or carry him over your shoulder on his belly or side. Because babies tend to turn their heads toward the center of the room or doorway, put your baby to sleep at alternate ends of the crib each night, and even change the position of the crib in the room occasionally. That way your baby will have to turn his head to look in a different direction when someone enters the room.

Encourage your baby to develop more neck strength by playing visual tracking games. When your baby is on his back, sit in front of him and lean your body slowly from side to side, talking to him so he'll keep watching you. He will be slow and his eyes will be jerky, and he might need you to help him move his head a little. When your baby reaches 6 to 8 weeks of age, play the same game when he is on his tummy. It's much more challenging and requires much more strength for an infant to track from side to side when on his tummy.

All of these frequent changes in head position encourage what we therapists call *range of motion* of the neck, which keeps the neck flexible and varies the spots where the skull gets pressure, thus reducing the risk of flat spots. An important reminder: your baby's favorite place to be is in your arms. Carrying your baby in your arms or wearing a front pack or backpack gets him off his head. As the same time, he is working on trunk and head control. The bonus? It provides a wonderful opportunity to bond and interact with your baby.

Variety Is the Spice of Life!

Add variety to your child's life! For healthy development, follow these suggestions for including various positions in your baby's daily routine during carrying, feeding, diapering, dressing, bathing, and sleeping times.

Carrying Time

Have fun as you carry your baby in a variety of positions. Babies learn to hold their head steady as they are held or carried in someone's arms. Approach and pick up your baby from different sides and consistently alternate the arm with which you hold him so he can turn and look to each side. Provide lots of head support to very young babies. Sitting them in your lap and letting their head bob is not a form of exercise— it is a sign that baby needs more support!

Activity #1: "I Can See Clearly Now" Carry

You can hold and carry your baby facing away from you to encourage visual exploration and tracking (the ability to follow a moving object using just the eyes). Position your baby's back against your chest and wrap one arm under his arms. Be sure to provide good support under baby's bottom using your other arm.

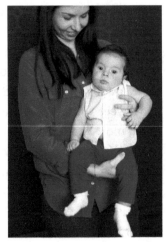

"I can see clearly now" carry

Activity #2: Football Hold With Head Support

Hold your baby in a belly-down position. One forearm should provide support to your baby's chest, and your hand will support your baby's head. Your other arm is positioned under your baby's trunk with your hand holding on to one thigh. Refrain from placing pressure on the chin or jaw area. This alternative carrying position is a form of tummy time.

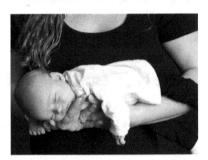

Football hold with head support

Activity #3: Football Hold

As your baby gains head control, try a traditional football hold. Hold him belly down on your forearm with his head resting near the inside of your elbow. Grasp his upper thigh with your hand and rest your other hand on his bottom. Hold your baby close to your body and this will help him

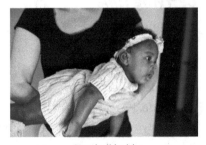

Football hold

feel safe and secure. Carrying your baby in this position encourages him to lift and turn his head to see what's going on around him, visually stimulating him.

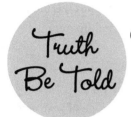

Truth Be Told

Carrying your baby in your arms frequently throughout the day requires your baby to use and strengthen his neck and trunk muscles and can help your baby enjoy being in a variety of positions.

Activity #4: Scoop Hold

With your baby in a sitting position, hold him with his back resting against the inside of your elbow, while holding his thigh with your hand. This is a comfortable position for your baby and it gives him a nice view of his surroundings.

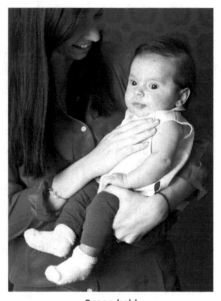

Scoop hold

Carrying your baby around helps him to build a tolerance for movement while increasing muscle strength and stimulating his movement system, which is important for developing balance, muscle tone, and visual skills. Make sure you feel confident with the positions in which you hold and carry your baby and try not to get too comfortable with one position. Remember, alternating positions encourages your baby to look in a variety of directions, which is good for stretching and strengthening the neck muscles. It's also good for you because varying the position in which you carry your baby can prevent muscle strain or injury to your back.

Feeding Time

During feeding, especially if your baby is bottle-fed, alternate the arm with which you hold your baby so he can turn and look to both sides. This also limits the pressure of your arm against the back of one side of baby's head. You can even feed your baby while he is on your lap facing you. Your baby's mouth should be in midline so it is lined up over his belly button.

Rather than always burping your baby in the traditional over-the-shoulder way, place him belly down on your lap for burping. Position him lengthwise across your lap with his arms over the edge of your leg and one hand on his bottom. Slightly elevate your thigh closest to your baby's head. As you burp him, be sure to turn his head to each side with a slight stretch. This ensures that the muscles in his neck are flexible and prevents any tightness.

When your infant can sit upright and use a high chair, always position the chair where he can easily see his surroundings and look to both sides. Spoon-feed him in the middle of his lips and to each side of his mouth to encourage balanced lip and jaw movements. Don't try to implement your infant's tummy-time routine immediately after feeding; this could cause discomfort due to pressure on the stomach, possibly causing him to spit up. No fun for you, and definitely no fun for him! However, if your infant sometimes spits up during tummy time, don't use that as an excuse not to do it. Being on his tummy will help his muscles get stronger, including those muscles that start to help him keep his feedings down. For some infants, supervised tummy time entails a little spit-up.

Diapering, Dressing, and Bathing Times

For diaper changes, occasionally alternate the side of the changing table on which you place baby's head. Remember to make a routine out of tummy time by rolling baby over on his belly after every diaper change. Having a schedule makes it easier to remember tummy time, and your baby will likely come to anticipate the routine. Just remember to never leave your baby's side during tummy time on the changing table. Use the safety strap and keep your hands on him at all times so there's no chance he'll roll off this high surface.

When dressing your baby, don't forget to include all of the lifting, carrying, and positioning suggestions provided thus far. You can even position him on his tummy or side while opening and closing fasteners located on the back of his clothing. After bathing, towel him off while

American Academy of Pediatrics Recommends Avoiding Sleep Positioners

Because your new baby spends so much time sleeping, it is important to be aware of safety measures while he slumbers. A sleep positioner is a flat or wedged mat with bolsters on either side that is frequently used to keep a baby positioned on his back while sleeping. These products have been on the market for more than 20 years, and many manufacturers claim they improve a baby's food digestion, reduce colic or the symptoms of gastroesophageal reflux disease, and may prevent positional skull deformities, although these claims have not been supported by research. The American Academy of Pediatrics (AAP) and US Food and Drug Administration (FDA) urge parents not to use these devices because a baby can suffocate while in a positioner. A baby can also become trapped and suffocate between the sleep positioner and the side of baby's bed. Unfortunately, sleep positioners are still on the market, despite these warnings from the AAP and FDA. Please be aware that the risk of suffocation is not worth any potential benefits, and don't be tempted to use a sleep positioner with your baby. Stick with AAP policy: put baby down for sleep on a firm, flat surface. Also, speak to your child's pediatrician if your baby has congestion or reflux.[65]

he's on his stomach. These are great ways to slip a little tummy time into baby's routine!

Sleeping Time

During the early weeks after birth, your newborn will spend most of his time sleeping. In fact, the average newborn sleeps 16 to 18 hours a day!

Remember to always position your baby on his back to sleep on a firm surface until he is at least 1 year old. Keep any soft or loose bedding, pillows, and stuffed animals away from baby's sleeping area, and never position him for sleep or play on beanbag chairs, waterbeds, memory foam, or other soft furniture.

As previously mentioned, alternate at which end of the crib your baby's head is positioned. Place your baby with his head at the opposite end of the crib each night. It may be helpful to keep a calendar near the crib, marking when you put his head at one end and the other. Observe the direction he holds his head during sleep. If it's consistently turned to one side after he's been sleeping for at least 15 minutes, turn his head to the opposite side. Then after a period, rotate his head to a straight-up position.

If your little one has a difficult time falling asleep, play classical music to soothe, calm, and relax him. Keep the volume low; there's a good chance the melody will lull him to sleep.

With early detection in most children, occipital plagiocephaly may be corrected with simple repositioning techniques along with stretching exercises. Remember, if your baby has a preferred head orientation, it may indicate the presence of one-sided neck muscle tightness. A physical or occupational therapist can address this with a stretching and positioning program. If your infant is younger than 1 year and has a moderate to severe flat spot, consult with your child's pediatrician. In certain cases, your child's pediatrician may refer you to a cranial band specialist (ie, an orthotist or occupational or physical therapist who specializes in this area). The terms *cranial band, cranial orthotic,* and *helmet* have come to be interchangeable. This process is called cranial remolding. The helmet is made of plastic and gently molds a baby's head back

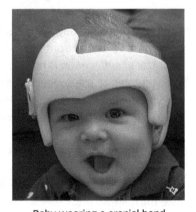

Baby wearing a cranial band

into place. How? It restricts skull growth in certain areas while allowing growth in other areas. It is typically worn for 23 hours a day, only to be removed for bathing and hair washing. Don't worry about your child's discomfort; wearing the helmet isn't painful, and the vast majority of babies do not even realize that it has been placed on their head.

The specialist follows up every 1 to 3 weeks to adjust the shape of the helmet. Treatment can take from 2 to 6 months. A molding helmet is frequently used along with occupational or physical therapy, which includes positioning and stretching exercises and education on daily routines that support head shape and development. The treatment program requires a strong commitment from parents to ensure directions are followed, adjustments are made, and therapy is adhered to. Please note that helmet therapy must always be carried out under the supervision of a physician. The US Food and Drug Administration requires that cranial bands be 510(k) compliant and approved. If at all possible, you will want to work with providers who have a high level of experience and can show you many before and after photos of babies they have personally treated.

Activities for Stretching Neck Muscles[66]

The following simple exercises and stretches are easy to carry out and will help keep your baby's neck and upper body flexible. Please remember that each exercise can be adapted to meet your baby's specific needs. All babies progress differently with their skills, and even babies who don't have tight neck muscles or plagiocephaly can benefit from these activities because they promote muscle development, strength, and flexibility. Plus, they offer a fun, healthy opportunity to bond with your baby.

You can use a 45-centimeter exercise ball for several of the following stretches. A 16-inch peanut ball also works nicely. You can purchase these at sports stores or many department stores. (Always use caution when using the ball; never take your hands off your baby during these activities.)

Before beginning, let your baby spend some time around the ball. Because the exercise ball is bigger than your baby, it may frighten him. Give him time to watch you playing with the ball and let him touch and pat it with your guidance.

Once you sense that your little one feels comfortable around the ball, you can move forward with the following exercises. If he resists the stretches, introduce them gradually. It may be helpful to have another person distract your child as you are working on the exercises. Also try playing games, singing songs, making funny faces, and blowing bubbles. You may even want to try the stretches while your baby is asleep. If so, make sure your child has been sleeping for at least 15 minutes before starting. This usually works best after he's fallen asleep in your arms.

Remember, if your baby has been diagnosed with torticollis or you suspect tight or shortened neck muscles, take him to see a physical or occupational therapist before doing these.

Ball Stretches

Your infant must be able to hold his head up independently to do these ball stretches.

Activity #1: On-the-Ball Stretch

Place your infant sitting upright on top of the ball facing away from you while you are kneeling or sitting behind the ball. His legs should be slightly separated. Place your hands on his hips for stability. Slowly and gently roll the ball forward. As you're doing this, baby may stabilize himself with his arms and hands, and he should naturally bring his head to an upright position. This exercise provides a nice stretch.

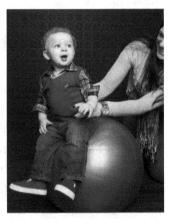

On-the-ball stretch

Activity #2: Side Ball Stretch

While your infant is still seated on the ball and facing away from you, roll the ball in the direction that he tends to turn his head. Keep your hands on your little one's hips as he uses his hands for stabilization. He should tilt his head, working to keep it in an upright position as you are moving the ball. This provides another nice stretch for tight neck muscles.

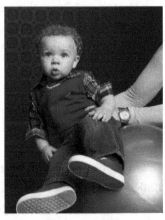

Side ball stretch

Activity #3: Tummy Ball Stretch

Next, position your infant on his tummy over the ball facing away from you. Sit behind the ball and hold his hips for stability. Slowly and gently roll the ball forward toward the floor. He will use his neck muscles to pull his head up. You can do this exercise in front of a mirror to encourage your baby to look up, or have someone sit in front of him to distract him. You can also roll the ball side to side, which works on the neck stretch. This exercise is good for your infant's balance skills and movement system.

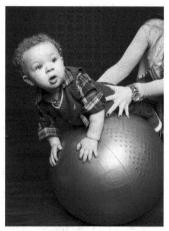

Tummy ball stretch

Bed Stretches

Activity #1: By-Your-Side Stretch

Lay your baby on his back on a firm bed. Sit in front of him at his feet, lean over him, and gently cradle the left side of his head with your right hand. Place your left hand on his chest. Gently turn his head toward his right shoulder, being sure to not put pressure on his chin. Hold this position for 5 seconds, and then do the same on the opposite side. If your baby resists you holding his head, shake a rattle or hold a musical toy to each side of his face and let him initiate the head turning by following the moving rattle. Once he starts turning his head, you may need to gently place your hand on the side of his head to help him hold the position. There's a good chance he won't mind because he'll be distracted by the rattle or toy. If he cries and resists your holding his head to the side, stop after a few seconds and try later. If your baby is unable to turn his head fully to one side, consult your child's pediatrician.

Activity #2: Up-and-down Stretch

Lay your baby on his back on a firm bed. Shake a rattle or hold a musical toy above his head and let him initiate tilting it upward, providing a nice stretch for his neck and jaw muscles. Slowly move the toy in the direction of your baby's feet. He should move his head downward as he follows the toy, eventually coming to a position where the chin is slightly tucked. Stop moving the toy before he lifts his head from the bed, and then repeat the stretch one more time.[67]

Tips **Ways To Prevent Occipital Plagiocephaly**

- Put baby to sleep on a firm, flat surface (on his back).
- Alternate your baby's head position by frequently placing him down for sleep at opposite ends of the crib. Occasionally change positions of the crib.
- Move the mobile to different ends of the crib.
- Alternate arms when holding and feeding your baby.
- Encourage supervised tummy time and side lying when baby is awake and supervised.
- Greatly limit the time your baby spends sitting in carriers and swings.
- If you notice your child consistently resists turning his neck to one side, consult with your child's pediatrician.

CHAPTER 6

Building a Solid Sensory-Motor Foundation: Birth to 3 Months

The wait is over—your baby has finally arrived! This is a thrilling time as you connect with your newborn and get to know one another. During this special time, you will develop a deep bond with your baby. The bonding that occurs between you and your newborn in these early days lays the foundation for your baby's ability to trust. Staying attentive to your baby's needs and remaining consistent in your caregiving lets your little one know she's accepted and loved unconditionally. By carefully reading your baby's cues and responding appropriately, you will support her development and learning.

A fun way to bond with your baby is through play. This chapter provides a variety of stimulating play activities and positions. Carrying out these activities will help you build a secure connection with your baby while supporting her development. As you incorporate the following activities into your everyday routine, you and your baby will have lots of fun together:

Developmental Milestones: Newborn to 3 Months

Look for your baby to display the following skills during this early phase of growth:

- Has basic reflexes such as sucking and rooting at birth.
- Closes fingers around a toy placed in hand at birth.
- Holds hands in fists in first month.
- Head falls back if not supported at birth.
- Brings hands to mouth.
- When on tummy, holds head up 45 degrees and bears weight on forearms.
- Developing head control.
- Brings hands together.
- Begins to hold hands open by 3 months.
- Swipes at objects.
- Grasps and shakes toys.
- Holds bottle for 1 minute.

Toy Tips: Newborn to 3 Months

The following toys are appropriate for facilitating baby's development during this age range. Always remember that these items should never be left in the crib with your baby when she is sleeping.

- Mobile with contrasting colors
- Rattles
- Wrist and ankle rattles
- Baby-safe mirror
- Colorful plastic keys
- Nursing pillow
- Soft books
- Music box

When your baby is awake, it's important to carve out time for play—it provides endless opportunities for fostering your little one's development. Babies experience the world firsthand through play, whether by shaking a rattle, manipulating a toy, or bouncing on your knee to music. Any activity a baby participates in that doesn't involve eating, hygiene, or sleeping can be classified as playtime.

During baby's early months, playtime should include proper positioning, familiarizing your child with the environment, and encouraging exploration. You may notice that most of the activities in this chapter focus on positioning. That's because the more positions your baby experiences throughout the day, the stronger her muscles will be, and strong muscles provide a solid developmental foundation. As you play with your baby in the various positions, she will enjoy your loving touch and the social interaction as you engage with her. Keep in mind that many of the positions and activities included in this chapter will also be appropriate to carry out with your baby after she is older than 3 months.

Emerging Skill: Visual Control

From the first days of your newborn's life, she will use her vision to explore her new surroundings. Your baby doesn't have full control of her eye muscles in the first few weeks, so her eyes may move in a jerky manner. They may not seem to be working together and may occasionally cross, but that's normal. Also, your baby's vision is somewhat blurry in these early days, so if you introduce toys with distinct shapes and high contrast, she will see them better. Because your baby can't focus on nearby objects yet, be sure to hold all toys 8 to 10 inches from her face during play, and only introduce one toy at a time.

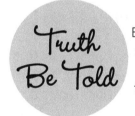

Babies are attracted to novel objects in familiar spaces, so occasionally change things in the environment, such as adding a new decorative item to the nursery, to catch your baby's attention.

Remember, however, that too much visual stimulation can be frustrating and may even cause your baby to become agitated. Because your baby's visual system is adjusting to this big new world, keep in mind that less is more. Keep the nursery simple and avoid an overabundance of wall hangings or decor that might be visually overwhelming for your baby.

Portable Rocking Sleeper: Limit to 30 Minutes a Day

The portable rocking sleeper has become popular in recent years. Many parents love these sleepers because they're easy to move from room to room and fold conveniently, saving space. Many parents report that this product helps their babies sleep more soundly and longer. However, the convenience of this product isn't worth the negative effect that its overuse can have on your baby. The current American Academy of Pediatrics (AAP) sudden infant death syndrome policy recommends back sleeping as well as a firm, flat mattress; these products do not fall within AAP safe sleep guidelines. Also, anytime young babies are placed on an incline and harnessed with their chin tucked, legs bent into flexion, and peripheral vision blocked, they are much less likely to work out any neck or head shape issues they may have been born with. If you have one of these sleepers, I recommend your baby spend no more than 30 minutes a day in it. That gives you just enough time to empty the dishwasher or fold a load of laundry. However, never use it for a break longer than 30 minutes.

Truth Be Told

You want to be sure that your baby is warm and snug, but don't be tempted to use bedding, blankets, and pillows when she is sleeping. Loose items such as these are a suffocation risk. Use a tight-fitting sheet on the mattress and dress baby in one-piece footed sleepers.

Activities: Newborn to 3 Months

The following activities are beneficial for your baby at this early age:

Activity #1: Go Mobile

Because baby's vision and hearing are developing quickly during the first few months after birth, one suggestion is a fun, bright mobile above the crib. Make sure the mobile has contrasting colors, such as red, black, and white, which will stimulate vision and focus. No doubt your baby will find the mobile interesting, and watching the moving objects is good for her visual tracking skills. A mobile that also plays music provides entertainment and enhances your baby's listening skills. When baby is looking at the mobile, be sure to point out the different colors and shapes. Turn the mobile on occasionally when baby is alone in the crib to provide visual and auditory stimulation. Rotate the mobile to a different position every so often so baby has a different view, as babies love novelty. This also encourages her to turn her head in different directions, which keeps her neck flexible.

Homemade Toy *A Unique Themed Mobile*

A homemade hanging mobile can be a special addition to the nursery. If your baby's room has a particular theme, incorporate the theme into the design of the mobile. A large, circular, wooden embroidery hoop makes a good frame, or you can use 2 or 3 tiers of wooden dowels with items hanging from each dowel. Mobiles should be fun and decorative as well as visually interesting for baby. You can hang a number of different items from the mobile. Colorful origami birds, boats, or flowers are options, as are knitted shapes or handmade stuffed animals. However, keep it simple—limit it to 3 to 4 hanging items so baby doesn't get visually overwhelmed. Use short lengths of ribbon, string, yarn, or sturdy fishing line to hang items from the mobile.

A good friend of mine made an amazing bird mobile, starting with 3 small tree branches. She tiered the branches about 6 inches apart using colorful embroidery thread and tiny eye hooks, then attached various colorful, hand-sewn birds to each of the sticks. It was a perfect addition to her bird-themed nursery!

When your mobile is complete, be sure to suspend it from a firmly mounted hook above baby's bed or tack it securely to the wall.

You may find that your baby falls asleep more easily if you remove the mobile from the crib at bedtime. Mobiles are great fun for play but may prove to be a distraction when it's time to slumber.

Mobiles intended for a baby's crib are designed for early development and are recommended from birth until 5 months of age. Once baby can sit, pull up, or get into a hands-and-knees position, it's time to remove it, or she could get entangled. If there is space, hang it on the nursery wall out of baby's reach for decor, or store it in a safe place for baby number 2.

Activity #2: It's Never Too Early to Read

Your baby's first exposure to reading will likely occur when you are interacting with her. Research suggests that reading books to your baby during the early months after birth will result in early reading skills. Plus, reading to your baby can be relaxing for you and soothing for her. The earlier you start, the better. Believe it or not, if you feel up to it, you can begin reading to your newborn while you are both still in the hospital. Reading is also a wonderful activity for a spouse or partner to carry out with baby. Be enthusiastic, using silly, animated voices and exaggerated faces to keep your baby's attention. Continue this wonderful habit into the toddler years and it's likely you will cultivate a love of reading in your little one. Reading exposes your child to language and increases knowledge.[68] Think about it—many of the smartest and most interesting people you meet in life are avid readers!

Story time encourages active listening skills and promotes concentration, and it's a wonderful way to stimulate your baby's mind. Many types of books appropriate for babies are available, including board, scratch-and-smell, lift-a-flap, and textured books. Engage your baby as you read through each book by pointing to and naming the details of each picture. You can even guide baby's hand to touch the pictures as you name them. This is a concrete way to help your child understand that the words you are saying are related to the pages in the book. With simple picture books, add the language component by explaining and describing what is happening on each page. For example, talk about facial expressions by saying, "Look, the girl is smiling. She must be happy," or, "Oh my, that boy is crying. He is sad!" Describe actions and concepts by pointing to a picture and telling your baby, "The baby is crawling under a table," or "The dog is jumping through a hoop." An animated voice with various inflections will keep baby interested.

Reading to baby is a wonderful way to liven up playtime while facilitating language. Plus, you're providing positive stimulation and increasing opportunities for the 2 of you to bond.

The Power of Nursery Rhymes, Rhythm, and Song

While you are reading to your baby, go ahead and include a nursery rhyme. Research tells us that nursery rhymes teach little ones about language, so this book includes a variety of old-fashioned songs and rhymes that will strengthen your baby's emerging language skills while introducing rhythm and patterns.

Interestingly, there is evidence that when a child learns nursery rhymes, poems, and songs early in life, this enhances her understanding of words and rhymes, which positively affects future vocabulary, reading, and spelling skills. Singing lullabies and reciting nursery rhymes is a lovely way to spend time with your baby, and the old rhymes might even bring back some of your own fond childhood memories.[69,70]

Activity #3: Happiness Is Tummy Time on a Blanket

In the first days of your baby's life, you can spread out a blanket or mat and play with her on the floor. Remove any loose items such as pillows or plush stuffed animals that might block baby's mouth or nose and cause problems with breathing. Before the play session, make sure she is happy and comfortable, never hungry or irritable. Position your newborn on her tummy with her elbows tucked to her sides. Start with only 15 to 20 seconds in this position, as baby's muscles have not yet gained strength. Your baby will alternate lifting her head with resting it on the supporting surface. Gradually

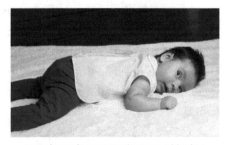

Happiness is tummy time on a blanket

increase the length of each tummy-time session as baby gets stronger. Her little forearms and hands should bear a portion of her body weight when she's on her tummy. While this activity strengthens the neck and trunk muscles, baby's hands and arms are getting a workout as well. In these early days, it's more important to provide frequent but brief tummy-time sessions throughout the day than 1 or 2 long sessions.

Activity #4: Knees-Tucked Tummy Time

Another option for newborn tummy time is to position baby on her tummy with her elbows bent and tucked next to her sides and her hips and knees bent and positioned underneath her. Your baby is basically in a fetal position. You may need to roll up several soft receiving blankets and tuck them around her bottom and legs to keep her stable. Talk to your baby and try to get her to lift her head and turn it from side to side.

When baby is holding her head up for a brief time, hold an interesting item such as a soft doll just above her eye level to attract her attention. The facial features of a doll will interest your little one and motivate her to hold her head up. Once the baby focuses on the doll, slowly move it from one side to another and then up and down and look closely to see if your baby watches it move. Remember, toys should be fairly quiet and presented slowly at this age so baby doesn't become overstimulated or frustrated. Try to finish the tummy-time session before she gets fussy, as it's best to finish on a positive note.

Activity #5: You've Really Got a Hold on Me

To improve your baby's head control, lay her on her back facing you, on the floor or your lap. Place your hands behind her with your palms supporting her shoulders and your fingertips supporting her head. Gradually raise her toward you, up into a sitting position. If your baby enjoys the motion, repeat several times. As she gets older and stronger, you can gently pull her into a sitting position just by holding her hands. However, do not transition to holding only her hands until she holds her head up well and can help by pulling herself up using her shoulders and arms.

For a happy distraction, add music to playtime. Be attentive to your baby's emotional communication and respond by playing appropriate music. If baby seems stressed or unhappy, play calming music; if baby is happy and engaged, you may want to introduce more playful music. One of baby's favorite sounds is mother's voice, so don't be shy—sing a lovely melody to your little one and watch the delighted response you receive. Your baby will especially enjoy music as you hold and carry her around because this adds movement to the mix.

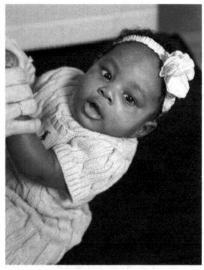

You've really got a hold on me

Activity #6: Hound Dog Puppet Play

Sock puppets are adorable and easy to make; without a doubt, your baby will enjoy puppet play! To create a simple sock puppet, you need a clean white sock and red and black fabric pens. Place your hand inside the sock and use your thumb and fingers to form a mouth. Use the black fabric pen to draw the eyes, nose, and ears (floppy puppy ears are cute), and use the red pen to draw a tongue inside the mouth. Be sure to color it in! The black and red provide a contrast against the white sock so your baby can see the puppet more clearly. This will help to develop her visual skills.

Position your baby on her side. She can be on the floor or in your lap. You may need to use a small pillow or rolled-up towel to give her some support behind her back, or use your leg as a support. If necessary, fold a small hand towel or burp cloth and place it under

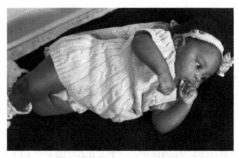

Side lying for a puppet show

baby's head like a pillow, or provide head support with your hand. Make sure her bottom arm is positioned in front of her in a comfortable position. It's time for a puppet show!

Truth Be Told

The sense of touch begins developing prenatally, and it is through touch that your baby will begin learning about herself and her surroundings. And there are many more benefits to touch! When you and your baby have skin-to-skin contact, you both release a hormone called *oxytocin*. Oxytocin, often referred to as the "love hormone," decreases stress, improves breastfeeding, and facilitates bonding between you and your baby.[71]

Tip **Set a Regular Bedtime Routine**

Research suggests that establishing a regular bedtime routine for babies helps them fall asleep more quickly and increases the duration of their sleep.[72]

Establish a bedtime routine when your baby is a newborn and your life will be easier in the long run. It provides a gentle transition from the busy day to the calmness of sleep. A regular routine such as rocking baby, reading a story, and a good-night kiss is a great way to prepare her for slumber time.

With the puppet on your hand, move it up and down and back and forth, keeping it within baby's line of vision. Make the puppet do a silly dance and sing silly songs. You can even have the puppet give her kisses! The more animated your voice and the more fun you are having, the more your baby is likely to enjoy it.

The Value of Baby Massage

Research reveals that touch is soothing and important for baby's development. When a parent massages a baby, this communicates to the baby that she is cherished and loved, which leads to a special connection between the 2 of you. Massaging your baby on a daily basis also has additional advantages. Research has shown that massage calms a baby, improves sleep, and reduces stress.[73,74] There are even training courses that instruct parents in baby massage techniques. Baby massage can begin as early as 2 to 3 weeks of age, or earlier if your child's pediatrician gives the approval. Use the following guidelines if you are unable to find a convenient training course:

Dim the lights and be sure the room is warm. Lay your baby, wearing only a diaper, on her back on a soft towel. Rub your hands together to warm them. Starting slowly and gently with her forehead, use gentle circular strokes to massage her temples, face, and jaw area. Slowly move down to her neck and shoulders, continuing to massage with gentle pressure. Avoid tickling your baby. Watch her closely and she will communicate if she's uncomfortable. If she seems fretful or turns her head away it may be time to stop and try later. If she is content and enjoying the massage, work your way down each arm to her hands. Rub her little palms, providing gentle pressure.

Roll baby gently over onto her back. Using circular strokes, rub the back of her head and move your way down her back and spine. Work your way around the rib cage using both hands. Continue to baby's bottom, thighs, lower legs, feet, and toes. Your baby will especially enjoy the massage if you sing, play soft music, and talk to her in a soothing voice. When you finish, your little one should be totally relaxed and possibly on the threshold of falling asleep!

Babies who have problems sleeping can benefit from massage. The pressure from the massage soothes the muscles and slows down the baby's heart rate and breathing, leading to a more restful night's sleep.

Before a baby ever leaves the womb, she is immersed in a sensory-rich environment. In a sense, a mother's womb massages the baby's body, providing a warm, soothing experience. Massage is comparable to the womb because it provides a calming setting while stretching and stimulating your baby's muscles. It can play an important role in healthy growth and development. No words can describe the benefits of your loving touch on your baby; therefore, I highly recommend all parents and caregivers learn the art of baby massage.

Emerging Skill: Head Control

At birth, your baby lacks head control because her neck muscles are relatively weak and her head is quite large compared with the rest of her body. At this stage, when holding and carrying your baby, it's important to provide head support at all times. As baby holds her head up for brief periods, she's strengthening her neck and back muscles. Tummy time also helps her develop head control. After 3 months, you will notice a great deal of improvement in your infant's ability to hold up her head, and around 6 months, head control will be strong and steady.

Baby Carriers: Use Only When Necessary

Baby carriers are extremely popular among new mothers. A carrier is typically part of a portable car seat system, which also includes a car seat base and stroller base. The carrier snaps into both base systems. They are quite convenient, as a new mother can buckle her baby into the carrier, walk out to the car, snap the carrier into the car seat base, drive to the park, remove the carrier, snap it into the stroller base, and take baby for a walk. But think about what this baby has missed out on! Typically, her mother would have held baby in her arms and carried her to the car. She would have placed baby in the car seat, then removed her and put her in the stroller. All the while, baby is enjoying mother's loving touch and using muscles in her trunk and neck while being held.

The portability and convenience of the carrier are appealing to busy parents, but as you can see, there are good reasons to limit the use of carriers. When in a carrier, many babies tilt their head to one side, which is not good for the neck and spine and can put pressure on one area of baby's head, possibly leading to a flat spot. Of course, brief periods in a carrier are not a problem, but if baby has a lot of travel time in her schedule, it's important to give her occasional breaks from the seat and to limit the amount of time she spends in other types of baby gear for the remainder of the day.

Safety Tip

Always fasten the safety straps when your baby is positioned in a carrier.

Many parents attach toys from the handle of a baby carrier so they dangle down, hanging several inches from the baby's eyes. As I have shared, babies can easily get too much visual stimulation, especially newborns. Unfortunately, parents may assume that baby is content and happy and continue to leave her there overstimulated. This can be very frustrating for baby! It is also important to remember that toys should never be attached to a car safety seat while in a moving vehicle because this poses a safety hazard.

Consider removing the dangling toys every so often, and if you are sitting with your baby, watch her carefully. After she plays with the toys for a while, if she turns her head to the side or shut her eyes, that may be her way of telling you, "I'm all finished here!"

Mothers should note that baby carriers can weigh up to 10 pounds, so when combined with the weight of a newborn, this can put a lot of strain on your back, shoulders, and arms. When possible, carry your baby rather than risking injury to yourself. Also, don't get into the habit of holding your baby on one side only. Rather, alternate arms to avoid placing undue stress on one side of your body.

Activities to Improve Head Control and Focus

The following activities provide alternatives to excess time spent in baby carriers, and many of them will improve your baby's head control:

Activity #1: Patty-cake

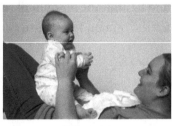

Lie on your back and slide your feet toward your hips so that your calves are near the backs of your thighs. You may need a pillow under your head for support. Sit your baby on your tummy facing you so that her back is resting against

Patty-cake

your thighs. Hold her hands with yours and gently clap them together to play a game of patty-cake.

❀ ❀

Patty-cake

Patty-cake, patty-cake, baker's man
(Take baby's hands through the motions.)
Bake me a cake as fast as you can
Roll it
(Roll her hands around each other.)
and pat it
(Clap.)
and mark it with a B
(Guide her finger to write a B in the air.)
And put it in the oven for baby and me!
(Kiss your baby!)

❀ ❀

Activity #2: Footloose

A wonderful movement experience for baby is for you to dance around while she's positioned over your shoulder. At an early age, gently support baby's head so it's lined up with her body. You can slowly dance around and sing to her while holding her in this position. She will enjoy the movement and at the same time will learn to tolerate the slight pressure against her tummy. Dance to all different types of music, including jazz, pop, and classical, depending on your baby's mood and whether you want to calm her down or pep her up. The movement is good for you and is also stimulating to baby's vestibular system. As your baby gets stronger and holds her head up, you won't have to provide as much support.

Activity #3: Heads Up, Baby!

Position your baby stomach down on your lap and slightly raise one of your legs above the other, providing a slight incline so baby can more easily lift her head. This position causes your baby to work against gravity to hold her head up and strengthens the neck muscles. At this early age, your baby will tire easily, so introduce this position gradually. Providing lap time allows baby to see what's going on around her, and if there's not enough excitement in the room, you can entertain her with a toy, rattle, or baby mirror.

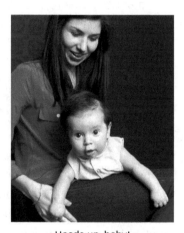

Heads up, baby!

Truth Be Told

Baby talk, also called "parentese," occurs when parents and caregivers instinctually speak to babies in an exaggerated, singsong, slow manner. This type of speech is critical to development because it helps babies pay attention to words and learn the various components of language.[3]

The Benefits of Babywearing

An alternative to transporting your baby via a stroller or carrier is babywearing. This is the practice of transporting a baby in a soft carrier that attaches to the caregiver's body. There are many benefits to babywearing. For example, research suggests that babies who are worn cry less, feel more secure, and bond with their caregivers as compared to babies who caregivers do not engage in babywearing.[75] Because the baby is in an upright position, there is a reduced risk of developing flat spots on the head. An added bonus to babywearing is that it frees up your hands, allowing for multitasking such as folding clothes, cleaning the house, or shopping. Additionally, one research study revealed that babywearing mothers respond more readily to their baby's cues than mothers who do not babywear, which promotes secure attachment.[76] Make sure that your baby is upright with nothing near the baby's nose and mouth that could interfere with breathing.

Activity #4: Peekaboo

Babies are typically delighted with games such as peekaboo and "gotcha." Lay baby on a blanket on the floor or bed and place a soft, folded washcloth or burp cloth under your baby's head for support. Position a small bolster pillow or rolled towel under your little one's thighs. This will slightly bend her hips and knees. This should be a nice, comfortable position for your baby.

Now sit directly in front of your baby. Cover your face using your hands or a scarf, then uncover your face and exclaim, "Peekaboo!" To play "gotcha," simply tell your baby, "I'm going to get you!" with your arms outstretched while wiggling your fingers and moving toward her. You can specify a body part you're going to get, such as, "I'm going to get your belly button," or, "I'm going to get your toes!" Lean forward and grasp baby gently or tickle her while saying, "Gotcha!" The more you laugh, kiss, and hug your baby, the more likely she will laugh with you.

While baby is on her back, add a bit of leg action to the activity. Gently grasp each of your baby's legs and guide them through walking or biking motions. Every so often, switch to baby's arms and guide them in a clapping motion. Baby will love the movement, and this is a great activity for body awareness.

Activity #5: Smiley Faces

Homemade smiley faces are simple to make and can be a fun way to entertain your little one! Using a black or red unscented marker, draw a smiley face on a white paper plate. You can also cut several different simple face patterns out of red or black construction paper and glue them onto paper plates. If you have access to a laminating machine, laminate them to keep them in good shape, or use sticky-back laminate. Hang the faces up on the wall next to the changing table to keep baby occupied while changing her diaper.

Another fun activity is to cut out large, basic patterns using black and red construction paper. Glue them on a small piece of poster board and laminate it or cover it with clear contact paper. Your baby will enjoy looking at circles, stripes, squares, crosses, and curvy lines. This is another option for baby to observe during a diaper change, or you may want to take it on a car ride and mount it in front of your baby's car safety seat. I did this and my little ones love it!

Homemade Toy Makeshift Rattle

Recycle a travel-sized mouthwash bottle and make a crafty rattle to stimulate your baby's vision and hearing. Remove the label from the bottle, clean it thoroughly, and allow it to dry completely. Fill the bottle halfway with colorful beads (Mardi Gras beads are a fun option; just snip the beads apart with a sturdy pair of scissors). Use nontoxic glue to secure the lid in place, giving the glue plenty of time to dry before using the rattle. Rattle play is wonderful for developing your baby's arm and hand skills, including reaching, grasping, and manipulating. Keep in mind when you make a rattle that it should be lightweight and easy for baby to grasp.

$\mathcal{T}ip$ *Swaddling Safely*

Your baby will feel safe and secure when swaddled in a blanket, but be sure that you swaddle her correctly. When a baby is swaddled too tightly, it is not good for her hip joints, and this could cause hip problems in the future. Be careful not to pull the blanket too tightly around baby's hips; leave plenty of space for her to move her legs and hips around.

When your baby is swaddled, take care that she does not get too warm, as this increases the risk of sudden infant death syndrome (SIDS). If your baby seems uncomfortable or unhappy with being swaddled, don't worry; swaddling may not be for her. Your baby will let you know what she likes and dislikes, so just follow her cues. She should always be positioned on her back when swaddled. Do not swaddle your infant at 2 months or older because there is a risk she will roll onto her side or stomach, which greatly increases the risk of SIDS.

Activity #6: Shake, Rattle, and Roll

If your baby is attempting to roll from her back to her stomach, this is a fun activity that will support her efforts. Begin by positioning her face up on a blanket. Hold her makeshift rattle about 6 inches above her chest and shake it to get her attention. When your baby reaches for the rattle, keep shaking while gradually moving it to the side opposite her reaching hand. Hold it just out of reach, and as she reaches toward the shaking rattle, this will initiate a roll. If baby is unable to roll over completely, gently grasp her hip or upper thigh on the side of her reaching hand and carefully guide her in rolling over the rest of the way. Once she's on her tummy, help her into a comfortable position by propping her up on her forearms.

Emerging Skill: Purposeful Movement

As the weeks pass, your infant gains more control of her movements. As we discussed in Chapter 2, gross motor development, or the ability to control the large muscles in the body, comes before fine motor development, which is the ability to manipulate the small muscles in the body. During this period in your baby's development, it's important to provide plenty of space for her to move her arms and kick her legs. She will enjoy watching her hands as she moves them about, and she may even bring her feet to her mouth for exploration. Provide plenty of opportunities for reaching, kicking, rolling, and exploring, as this is good for baby's motor skills.

Activity #7: Two Sides of the Same Coin

Encourage your baby to look at both of her hands. This will help her learn that she has 2 sides. Move one arm in front of her eyes, gently stretch and manipulate her fingers, and then do the same to the other side. Talk or sing to her about having 2 arms and hands during the activity.

Bumper Pads: Avoid Use According to the American Academy of Pediatrics

Parents often use bumper pads to keep babies from bumping their heads against the slats of a crib, but there is no proof that these products prevent serious injury. In fact, bumper pads are actually dangerous. You may be tempted to use a bumper pad, especially if your little one is rolling or scooting toward the slats of the bed while sleeping, but the AAP officially recommends that bumper pads never be used in cribs because of the potential risk of suffocation, strangulation, or entrapment.[77] If you have a bumper pad in your baby's bed, remove it immediately, but don't throw it away if you want to make the homemade tummy-time bolster described in the box later in this chapter.

Activities to Encourage Purposeful Movement and Bonding

These activities will help your baby develop muscles and coordination, and just as importantly, they provide wonderful opportunities to spend time with your little one.

Activity #1: Bring on the Bolster

Use the small homemade bolster, or roll up a thin towel or blanket into a bolster shape, and place it under your baby's chest. Position baby's arms over the roll with her hands stretching out in front of the roll. Baby's chin should still be positioned slightly in front of the roll so her mouth and nose get plenty of air. A low-profile nursing pillow also provides support during tummy time. If baby appears uncomfortable on the bolster or nursing pillow, try slowly rocking her side to side or gently patting her bottom while singing a tune. The movement and melody should help her tolerate being on her stomach for a longer period.

If your baby is not tolerating the position, put a baby-safe mirror in front of your little one so she can see herself, or lie down facing your baby and make eye contact with her. She will enjoy looking at your face, and this provides a perfect opportunity to connect and interact with her. Only use a bolster or nursing pillow occasionally during tummy time, as this doesn't work baby's muscles as much as basic tummy time on the floor.

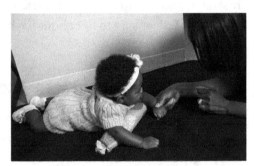

Bring on the bolster (Always provide supervision when using a bolster during tummy time.)

If baby is not lifting her head while positioned on her stomach on the floor, take your hand and press down gently on her lower back or bottom in the direction of her feet to shift the weight away from her upper body. This directs more of baby's weight toward her hips, making it easier for her to push up with her arms and lift her head.

Activity #2: Stuck on You

This activity is based on a task that was carried out in a research study at Kennedy Krieger Institute.[78] The 3-month-olds in the study wore mittens with Velcro strips during play that allowed them to grasp and move toys with Velcro strips. Allowing them to manipulate toys using the mittens increased the infants' interest in human faces, suggesting

Homemade Tummy-Time Bolster

Your baby will benefit from using a small bolster occasionally during tummy time, so why not upcycle that unsafe, unneeded bumper pad into the perfect baby bolster? Actually, go ahead and make 2 sizes because your baby will need an extra-small one in those early months and a larger size as she gets older. Only use your tummy-time bolster when your baby is awake and supervised.

Items needed include
- Bumper pad or old comforter
- Soft twine
- One upcycled sheet, pillowcase, or section of cotton fabric
- Decorative ribbon
- Needle and thread

For the small bolster, cut off an 18-inch strip of the bumper pad. Tightly roll the strip up diagonally so that the width is 12 inches and the diameter is approximately 4 inches. Take a piece of string, wind it around the bumper pad to secure it into the shape of a bolster, and tie the string in a secure knot. Cut the sheet, pillowcase, or fabric so that it's 4 inches wider than the 18-inch bolster on each side, and make sure that there is enough fabric to wrap around the bolster twice. You can use pinking shears or, if you have a sewing machine, a rickrack stitch around the edges of the sheet as the trim. Roll up the bumper pad bolster tightly inside the sheet and take 2 pieces of twine and secure each end tightly so the bolster looks like a piece of wrapped candy. Use the decorative ribbon and make small, pretty bows to cover the twine. The bolster is ready for tummy time!

For a larger bolster, just repeat the process with the same material, making the width approximately 18 inches and the diameter 8 inches.

a link between motor skills and social development. And hey, it sounds like lots of fun for your baby!

To make the mittens, you will need a pair of infant mittens (or baby booties) and sticky-back Velcro strips. Attach several short strips of Velcro loop to each of the mittens on the palm side near the fingertips.

Next, select one of your baby's toys that will fit into her palm and attach a hook strip of Velcro to it. A toy that rattles will be even more stimulating for your baby. It's time to play!

You can carry out this activity in any position that allows your infant to move her arms freely. One option is to hold her close against you in your lap sitting on one of your thighs. First, put the mittens on your little one's hands. If baby is on the right side of your lap, use your left hand to hold a toy in front of her within her reach so that it will stick to the mitten if she swipes it. Move the toy around and talk to your baby, encouraging her to get the toy. Once she swipes and the toy sticks to the mitten, watch your baby closely as she moves the toy around. Is she looking at her hands? Is she watching the toy? Give her time to make the connection that when she moves her arm, the toy also moves.

Store your sticky mittens in a convenient spot. You'll definitely want to let baby try this activity again.

Activity #3: Can't Smile Without You

While baby is positioned tummy down on the floor, you or an older sibling lie tummy down facing her. If she doesn't yet have good head control, provide assistance by gently lifting her chin so she can see your face. Your baby prefers a human face—especially yours—to other images! Closer to the end

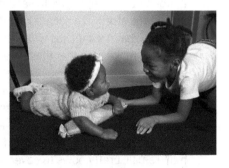

Can't smile without you

of her third month, she will be more social and enjoy any attention that comes her way. Attempt to get her to smile by sticking out your tongue, smiling at her, and making other funny faces. Who knows? You may even hear your infant's first giggle!

Activity #4: All Shook Up

Place your baby on her back on a blanket. Hold the wrist rattle and shake it on the right side of your baby's head, encouraging her to turn toward the sound. Now move the rattle to her left side and shake it again so baby turns in that direction. Your baby will be unable to control her grasp for several months, so the wrist rattle will come in handy. Attach the rattle to one of your baby's wrists like a bracelet, and she will be delighted when she moves her hand and it jingles. After a while, move the rattle to baby's other wrist. This wonderful tool helps your baby discover her hands, and it also teaches her about sound. With every wiggle of her arm, the rattle will jingle and stimulate baby's hearing. You can even attach it to her ankle to see how she responds! These rattles stimulate your baby's visual system because she will likely turn

Homemade Toy *Colorful Wrist and Ankle Rattles*

My babies loved rattles that fit on their wrists or ankles. I simply sewed a small rattle securely onto a small baby bootie, and we were in business! If you are more creative, you can sew a handmade wrist or ankle rattle using the following directions:

For this fun wrist rattle, all you need are
- Several scraps of sturdy, colorful cotton fabric
- A strip of half-inch–wide ribbon
- A pair of scissors
- Needle and thread
- Two medium-sized jingle bells
- Sew-on Velcro closures

Take several colorful scraps of sturdy cotton fabric and cut them into your favorite shapes using scissors. I prefer stars and moons. The shapes should be 1 to 1½ inches wide. Place the 2 sides of the shapes together with the wrong sides facing out and stitch the edges tightly together, leaving enough space to insert 2 small jingle bells. Turn the shapes right-side out, insert the jingle bells, add a small bit of cotton filling, and finish stitching the shape closed. Use a complimenting color of half-inch–wide ribbon to make the wristband. Determine the length by sizing it to your baby's wrist and add half an inch to each end of the wristband for the Velcro closure. Stitch the Velcro pieces to each end of the ribbon to make the strap. Stitch the jingle bell shape onto the center of the wristband, and you have your handmade wrist rattle. You did it!

Remember to always supervise your baby closely while she is playing with her homemade rattle.

her head to see the rattle when it moves. She is getting her first lesson on cause and effect!

Activity #5: Roll With It

When your baby begins to show an interest in rolling from her stomach to her back, you can carry out this activity to support her development. Sit in front of your baby during tummy time, hold her makeshift rattle to one side, and shake it. When she looks to that side, hold her at her shoulders and guide her through the motion of rolling from her stomach to her side. She may try to take over and finish rolling onto her back—that's great! Be sure to keep your hands on her shoulders just in case she needs assistance. Move slowly and be gentle during this activity. Let baby rest, and then repeat the activity to the opposite side if she is up for it. Remember, don't push your baby to master a skill. If she's not attempting to roll yet, wait and carry out this activity when she's ready.

Activity #6: Ticket to Ride

Your baby's head control should be improving. Once she's able to hold her head up for a brief period, hold her on your lap facing you while providing plenty of support to her upper body. Slowly raise her up, then back down, then gently raise her back up again. You don't want her to drop her head back, so give her head support if needed. Lean in close to her face and sing or make faces to keep her engaged. She will enjoy the movement as well as the interaction.

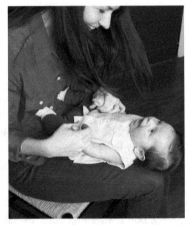

Ticket to ride

Activity #7: Back on Your Side

While your infant is positioned on her side, place one of your hands under her arm that is close to the floor and the other hand on her opposite hip. Slowly roll her over so that she's positioned on her belly.

After she spends some time on her tummy, gradually roll her so that she is in the side-lying position on the opposite side.

As Your Baby Grows So Do Her Needs

As you now know, it is important for your infant to spend time in a variety of positions throughout the day. Throughout the first year after birth, your baby will spend time in many different positions. For example, at 3 months, your infant will spend approximately half of her waking hours being held, and at this early age, she is totally dependent on you to change her position. Once she begins to sit independently, she will spend more time sitting, and when she begins to walk, she will spend much of her time in an upright position. As you can see, the positions that she experiences will naturally change as her motor skills develop, and being in a variety of positions will change how she interacts with the world. This will ultimately affect her opportunities for learning in a positive way![79]

Can you believe that 3 months have passed since your baby's birth? Time really does fly when you're having fun! You've supported your infant's growth and development by carrying out the activities suggested in this chapter, and you and your little one have shared special time together.

Bonding with your child is as critical to the developmental process as nutrition and physical activity. In fact, research demonstrates that infants use their emotions to guarantee their closeness to mom or dad.[80] What does that mean? When your baby wants you to come, she cries! That's her way of communicating with you, so it's important that you respond to her cries sensitively and consistently. Responding in this manner allows your baby to feel safe and secure and reinforces the connection between you. That bond becomes even stronger as you spend quality time together while participating in the activities suggested in this book.

CHAPTER 7

Enhancing Development With Retro Activities: 4 to 6 Months

From 4 to 6 months, your infant's sensory-motor skills develop rapidly, making this an exciting time for your little one. As he becomes more aware of his surroundings, he enjoys examining anything within his reach. This is a wonderful time to encourage reaching, grasping, batting, rolling over, and sitting up. Talk to your baby as frequently as possible during this phase because infants of this age listen carefully to every word you say! Slow down and enjoy the precious moments with your infant because it won't be long before independence reigns.

Developmental Milestones: 4 to 6 Months

Look for your infant to display the following skills during this 4- to 6-month phase of growth:
- Grasps toy crudely
- Brings both feet to mouth for play
- Raises head and chest when lying on stomach
- Reaches out for toy
- Picks up rattle
- Holds rattle
- Grasps and holds a cube
- Holds small toy with both hands
- Rolls from stomach to back
- Rolls from back to stomach
- Grasps tiny toy with palm and fingers
- Holds one toy in each hand

Toy Tips: 4 to 6 Months

The following toys are appropriate for facilitating your infant's development during this age range. Remember that these items should never be left in the crib with your infant when he is sleeping.

- Colorful plastic keys
- Wrist and ankle rattles
- Plastic rings that link
- Textured toys
- Cloth or vinyl books
- Baby-safe mirrors
- Soft stacking blocks
- Soft stacking rings
- Soft 10- to 14-inch ball
- Noisemaking toys such as small rattles or maracas
- Large connectable beads

Toy Selection Tips

Choose age-appropriate toys.	Be sure to check the package for the recommended age range for any toy. Toys that are above an infant's age level may pose a safety hazard because of small parts on which your infant could choke.
Think manipulative.	Toys that can be manipulated, such as shape sorters, stacking blocks, and baby-safe puzzles, are great for an infant's fine motor, cognitive, and perceptual skills. Babies can have lots of fun while building important developmental skills.
Consider durability.	Consider how well the toy is going to hold up over time. Is it washable, well-constructed, durable, and safe?
Safety first!	Check for loose parts on all toys. Remember that long ribbons and strings are a safety issue. Be sure to keep all toys clean by wiping them down regularly.
Think multisensory.	Developmentally appropriate toys that are colorful and have different textures will grab an infant's attention and stimulate his senses. Toy musical instruments, textured puzzles, mobiles, and baby-safe mirrors are excellent multisensory options.

As a parent, it is nice to know that there are lots of options for supporting your infant's development and helping him reach his potential during this time. Use equipment wisely and have fun with the following activities, which will improve the strength, balance, and coordination your infant needs to master developmental milestones. Many of the positions and activities included in this chapter will also be appropriate to carry out with your infant when he is older than 6 months.

Emerging Skills: Batting and Visual Tracking

During the next few months, your infant's movements will become more intentional and controlled as he becomes even more visually interested in the world around him. He will begin to follow items with his eyes and actively use his arms to bat or swipe at various objects. These may look like random movements, but they are becoming more purposeful. If he hasn't already, he'll soon reach for and grasp items with success. What an exciting time of discovering a great big world!

Bouncer Seat: Limit to 30 Minutes a Day

On days when the laundry piles up or you have a ton of housecleaning to do, you may be tempted to plop your little one in a bouncer seat and let him entertain himself for a while, especially if he appears to be content in the seat. Most bouncer seats have dangling toys that manufacturers claim "encourage babies to reach, bat, swipe, tug, and enhance eye-hand coordination." Many infants will sit quietly, staring toward and occasionally batting at the toys hanging just in front of their eyes, which can keep them occupied for long periods. Because the hanging toys attached to the bouncer are stationary, simply watching them does nothing to improve your infant's visual tracking skills, and he may get overstimulated by toys hanging so close to his face. Also, when an infant is positioned in one of these devices for too long, active movement and exploration are limited, so don't give in to the temptation to overuse the bouncer seat.

If you have a bouncer seat, use it no more than approximately 30 minutes each day. When your infant contentedly sits in a bouncer within eyesight, you have the perfect opportunity to fold a load of clothes or sweep the kitchen floor. But after 30 minutes have passed, remove your little one from the bouncer. If possible, break up the time in the bouncer into two 15-minute or three 10-minute sessions.

Activities: 4 to 6 Months

Many of the activities listed here are good for your infant's eye-hand coordination. How? They require the muscles in your little one's eyes and hands to work together as he watches moving toys and swipes at them. These activities are also language-rich, meaning they include abundant opportunities for verbal and social interactions. Enjoy carrying out these activities with your infant.

Keep Your Baby Safe

Never place a bouncer seat on a table, sofa, countertop, or bed with your infant in it. The seat could fall from any elevated surface and injure him.

Activity #1: Puppet on a String

Tie one of your infant's favorite toys to a short piece of ribbon. (*Note:* Use caution with the ribbon, making sure it's only 3 to 4 inches long. Don't allow your infant to handle ribbon or string because it poses a choking risk.) Carefully position your infant on his back on a blanket and dangle the toy above his head, just within his arm's reach. Encourage him to reach up and bat at the toy to make it move. Take his hand and guide him through the motions on the first attempt if he doesn't take a swipe. Once he successfully strikes the toy, praise him by saying excitedly, "Good job! You touched the toy! Look—you made it move!"

Slowly move the toy from one side to another, then up then down, pausing occasionally to give your infant the chance to reach in different directions and swipe at it. Be sure to praise your little one every time

Homemade Toy *Baby Bootie Rattle*

How many times have you finished a load of laundry only to discover you're missing one of your baby's booties? Fortunately, you no longer have to discard the extra bootie. You now have a fantastic way to upcycle it into an adorable baby rattle. To make it, you'll need

- A cute, colorful baby bootie
- Cotton batting
- Two small jingle bells
- Colorful ribbon
- An empty, childproof, travel-sized, cylinder-shaped acetaminophen or ibuprofen bottle

Place the jingle bells inside the childproof bottle and secure the top in place. Stuff the batting tightly into one end of the baby bootie, then add the bottle with the jingle bells inside. Now stuff the other end of the bootie with batting, tuck in the open edge of the bootie (rounding it at the corners to match the toe end of the bootie), and stitch it together neatly. Take the ribbon and wrap it tightly around the center of the bootie over the cylinder-shaped container so you make a handle for the rattle. Tuck the end of the ribbon out of sight and stitch it securely in place.

he successfully connects with the toy. This activity exercises eye-hand coordination, addresses visual tracking skills, and stimulates language. A noisemaking toy such as a rattle adds even more fun to the mix—and it's one you can make yourself.

Activity #2: Shake It Up, Baby

At around 4 or 5 months of age, your infant will start to move his eyes without turning his head. This is the beginning of visual tracking, which is the ability to follow moving objects with smooth, coordinated eye movements. This game helps improve visual tracking skills needed for the future skills of reading and writing. The ability to visually focus also improves during this period, so be sure to incorporate play that encourages focusing and tracking. Here's an example.

While your infant is lying on his back, hold a rattle approximately 10 inches away and shake it. Once your baby focuses his eyes on the rattle, move it up and down, giving him time to follow it with his gaze. Bring the rattle back to the middle, then take it slightly to the left and right. All the while, carefully observe to see if your baby continues to follow the rattle with his eyes. If he happens to break his gaze, shake the rattle again to get his attention. (*Note:* You may need to gently support your infant's head to prevent him from turning his head to follow the rattle, and that's fine. For this particular activity, his head should remain still so that only his eyes move.)

After practicing visual tracking, you may want to encourage your infant to swipe or reach and grasp, as he did in the previous activity. Gently shake the rattle, positioning it within his reach at his midline. If he doesn't reach for it on his own but seems interested, give him guidance. When he does make contact with the rattle, praise him by saying, "Good! You touched the rattle!" Chances are he'll try to grasp the rattle, and if he does, let him have it. He'll probably hold it with one hand and manipulate or touch it with the other. That's great—he's using what we therapists call bilateral skills!

Activity #3: Chatting It Up

You can entertain your infant by communicating with him while he is lying on his back or in a position that doesn't require close supervision, talking to him as you are following through with your daily routine. If you are unloading the dishwasher, for example, you can tell him what you are doing by naming the colors of the dishes as you are putting them away; you could also count cans as you stock the pantry. It's simple to find natural teaching opportunities throughout your daily routine. Talk to your infant by naming the color of each piece of clothing while sorting laundry, describing what you are doing as you cook a meal, or counting plates and silverware as you set the table for dinner. Your infant is always listening to you and always learning. Every bit of information he takes in at this young age provides a foundation for future communication skills.

Activity #4: Crocodile Rock

Position your infant tummy down on your chest while holding him securely under his arms. Rock your body from side to side to incorporate movement. This can be a great way to calm him if he's not crazy about being on his tummy, and the rocking provides wonderful stimulation for the movement system. Talk or sing to him as you rock back and forth to keep him occupied. One of my favorite songs to sing while holding baby in this position is "Row, Row, Row Your Boat."

❖ ❖

Row, Row, Row Your Boat

Row, row, row your boat,

Gently down the stream.

Merrily, merrily, merrily, merrily,

Life is but a dream.

❖ ❖

Activity #5: Magic Carpet Ride

Spread a blanket on the floor and place your little one on it, tummy down. You can hold your infant's attention by selecting a blanket with bold, interesting patterns, such as contrasting stripes and different textures, to provide variety and stimulation. Better yet, create an activity blanket! To make it, scatter several colorful, interesting toys on an ordinary blanket. Make sure the toys fit nicely into your infant's hand if he attempts to grasp one of them.

This activity provides a wonderful opportunity for your little one to entertain himself for brief periods—a practice that can increase his attention span. It's good for him to spend time playing on his own, and it gives you time to work on a hobby such as knitting or reading, all the while keeping your eye on him.

If your infant gets restless, talk to him; if you're reading a book, occasionally read a passage aloud in an animated voice to keep him occupied. The content doesn't matter as long as you're animated and change your voice inflection while reading. Your infant will enjoy the experience.

You can even do your own exercises during your infant's independent floor play. For example, sit near your infant on a mat and do sit-ups, push-ups, and leg lifts. Your motion will hold his attention and entertain him. Occasionally say what you're doing to bring in some language. All the while, your infant gains muscle strength from being positioned on his tummy; plus, it's another opportunity to take pressure off his head. (*Note:* Be sure to keep a close eye on your infant the entire time you're exercising.)

Activity #6: Pull Out That Scarf!

Babies love colorful scarfs, so don't throw yours away when they wear out or go out of style. You'll need a paper towel roll or cardboard tube from a finished roll of gift wrap for this activity. Use a sturdy pair of scissors and cut the tube to 8 inches in length. Stuff a scarf inside the tube and show your infant how to pull out the scarf. Encourage him to push it back inside the tube and pull it through from the other side. Be sure to give him some help if he needs it.

You can also tie several scarves together and stuff them inside the tube or a larger recycled container. Your infant will enjoy pulling out the scarves and stuffing them back inside the container. Remember to praise him for his success!

Truth Be Told

Research reveals that the interactions children have with parents and caregivers early in life are extremely important. Positive interaction is an important part of the bonding process, and when a baby has a secure bond with one or both parents, he is likely to attain emotional and cognitive abilities more rapidly than a baby who is not secure in a primary relationship.[81]

Emerging Skills: Rolling Over, Strengthening, Balance, and Movement

Your infant is now initiating independent movement, rolling from his stomach to his back, among other moves. At about the 6-month mark, he'll likely learn to roll from his back to his stomach independently. Because rolling strengthens the neck, tummy, back, and hip muscles, it's a good idea to provide plenty of opportunities for him to roll.

Many infants love to be rocked, bounced, and moved about. Balance and movement play an important role in gaining the postural control and coordination they need to move their bodies about in space—to roll, scoot, crawl, and walk.

Around this age, when your baby is positioned on his back, you might see him reach with his right hand and play with his left foot or use his left hand to grab his right foot. This is called crossing the midline. You may be wondering what the term *midline* means. Visualize an imaginary line that runs from the top of your baby's head past his belly button to between his feet, dividing his body in half. That is his midline! When an infant crosses the midline, it means that the right and left sides of the brain are communicating with each other. If your infant isn't already reaching across his midline to grasp toys or other desired items, he will be doing so soon! The ability to cross the midline is important for future tasks such as drawing, reading, handwriting, and shoe tying.

Changing Table With Fewer Than 4 Sides: Avoid Use

Once your infant is able to roll over, if you are using a changing table with fewer than 4 sides, he could fall to the floor, leading to serious injury. The most recent safety standards require all changing tables to have 4 sides. To make it even safer, secure your infant to the changing table with a safety strap if one is available. Most importantly, never leave your infant's side, and hold on to him with one hand during a diaper change. Changing tables aren't recommended after your child reaches 2 years of age.

Activities That Address Core Muscles

The following activities are good exercise for your infant's core muscles, which make crawling and sitting up easier for your little one:

Activity #1: Little Piggy Game

"This Little Piggy" is a traditional, fun, and entertaining activity that's been around for years. It helps your infant understand where his hands, fingers, feet, and toes are located. As you play this game, you teach your infant about body awareness.

Start this game with your infant on his back, making sure to hold his feet up so he can see you wiggling his toes. Begin by holding and wiggling the big toe on one foot and saying the poem in an animated singsong manner.

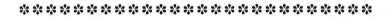

This Little Piggy

This little piggy went to market (big toe)

This little piggy stayed home (second toe)

This little piggy had roast beef (third toe)

This little piggy had none (fourth toe)

And this little piggy went wee wee wee all the way home (little toe)

Don't forget to give your infant a tickle at the end!

Once you've gone through the toes on one foot, move to the big toe on the next foot and repeat the rhyme. When you've finished with "This Little Piggy" on the toes, gently assist your infant in rolling from his back to his stomach. Place a rattle or another interesting toy in front of him, and when he sees it, move it over to one side, slightly above his head. As he watches you moving the toy, he will be motivated to roll toward the side where you're placing the toy; if he can't make it all the way over, gently grasp his upper thigh on the side opposite the toy and help him to roll onto his side, then over to his tummy. Now that he's in the tummy position, you're ready to play "This Little Piggy" with his fingers. Playing this game while he's positioned on his stomach strengthens neck, back, and upper body muscles, which will also make rolling over and sitting up easier for your baby.

Activity #2: Wheels on the Bus

For this activity, you will need your exercise ball. With him in front of you, place your infant over the ball stomach down, holding him at his hips. Roll the ball slowly back and forth several times. Watch closely to be sure your little one is enjoying the rocking sensation. This movement is good for his movement system; however, remember to always keep both of your hands on him the entire time to keep him safe. Add a little fun to the mix by singing "The Wheels on the Bus" as you roll your infant back and forth.

❊ ❊

The Wheels on the Bus

The wheels on the bus go round and round

Round and round, round and round

The wheels on the bus go round and round

All through the town

❊ ❊

Activity #3: Yakety-yak, Please Talk Back

Position your infant on your stomach or chest while you lie in a reclined position on a bed or in a reclining chair. The farther back you recline, the more effort it will take for your infant to hold up his head, which is a better workout for those neck and trunk muscles. Use a pillow to sup-port your head. In this position, your infant can see your face easily and will feel comforted by being nestled up against you. This is a fun time for interacting and socializing with your little one and playing imitation games, which are great for language and social skills. Encourage him to imitate sounds such as "ooh, ahh," and move on to "pa, da, ma" with time. Also, imitate your infant when he makes these sounds because this reinforces language interaction and speech development. By being at his eye level, you'll begin to understand the nonverbal communica-tion he directs toward you. This is similar to carrying on a conversation with your little one, but you're doing so in his language! This interac-tion will be stimulating and enjoyable for your infant, and the one-on-one time you spend interacting with him down at his level is so special. As you play with him like this, you are creating memories that you will always recall fondly.

Activity #4: Monkey See, Monkey Do

Spread out a blanket on the floor and lay you and your infant tummy down, facing one another. This is a wonderful position to play in with your infant and encourage him to imitate facial expressions and sounds.

You may be surprised at how he'll attempt to imitate your expressions as you stick out your tongue, smile broadly, click your tongue, or blow raspberries. Make each expression slowly, then give your little one plenty of time to attempt his imitation. Be sure to praise him when he imitates you successfully! Give him verbal feedback by saying, "Good job! You made a happy face just like Daddy did. Now can you stick out your tongue like this?" This activity not only teaches your infant to imitate; it's great for attention span and socialization skills.

Activity #5: Mustang Sally

Sit on the floor with your knees bent. Position your infant facing away from you and seated upright on your knees, holding him firmly under the arms or at the hips. Talk to your little one to reassure him that he's safe, telling him you're going to play the horsey game. Slowly move your legs side to side to provide movement. He should love this! Hum a tune and sing the lyrics to the horsey song as you move your legs. When you say, "Don't fall down," slide your feet forward!

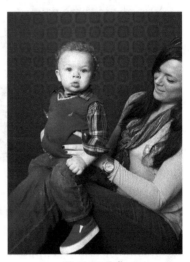

Mustang Sally

❖ ❖

The Horsey Song

Ride a little horsey

Down to town

Oops, little horsey

Don't fall down!

❖ ❖

Activity #6: Up Where You Belong

When you're in a reclined position with your knees bent and feet flat, have your infant sit upright facing you in your lap. Your infant's shoulders should be resting against your thighs. (You'll probably need a pillow under your head for support.) This is a perfect position to play, sing, and interact with your child. You can also work on language imitation skills. If he isn't holding his head up well, be sure his head stays properly aligned as it rests back against your thighs.

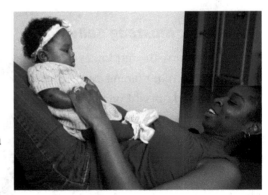

Up where you belong

After playing with your infant in this position for a while, extend your knees slightly, sliding your feet forward away from your bottom. This will lower him into a reclined position. Let him grasp your hands, then pull him back up to sitting while saying, "Up, up, up you go!" After he sits up for a moment, gently lower him against your thighs again, saying, "Down, down, down you go!" This improves his grasping skills and upper extremity and trunk stability, all while having fun!

When my children were babies, this became my favorite position to teach them animal sounds. I would name an animal, simulate the noise the animal makes, and describe several of the animal's traits, saying, "A horse is big, runs very fast, and says neigh, neigh!" Of course, another fun way to teach animal sounds is by singing the classic song "Old MacDonald Had a Farm" to your baby.

Activity #7: Cross Your Heart

Place a favorite toy in front of your baby on his right side and prompt him to reach for it using his left hand. Provide a bit of guidance if he needs it. Now repeat the activity, but have him reach across midline to his left side using his right hand. Be sure to cheer him on when he successfully grasps the toy!

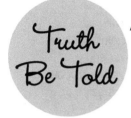

An infant's sleep pattern begins to normalize at around 6 months of age, but up until then, his sleep schedule will likely vary. In the early months, it's a good idea for parents to rest when baby sleeps.

Emerging Skills: Sitting Up, Reaching, and Grasping

Before your baby gains the trunk strength and head control to sit up independently, he may be able to prop sit. Prop sitting is when a baby sits upright and maintains his balance by leaning forward on both hands. Keep in mind that your baby may easily lose his balance when prop sitting and tumble over, so stay close by or surround him with pillows until he can maintain the position independently. You can also tuck a thin folded towel or receiving blanket under his bottom, which will shift his balance toward his arms and hands and help him stay upright.

As your little one nears the 6-month mark, his trunk control will continue to improve and he will likely begin to sit upright for brief periods. While sitting, he may reach for toys and grasp them, bring his hands together, and watch his hands as he moves them. He may even begin to move his fingers individually, but he won't yet have control of these movements.

Sitting up is a great time to practice reaching and grasping skills. As your infant watches himself reach, grasp, and bring items to his mouth, his balance and eye-hand coordination improve. Having strong trunk muscles provides a solid foundation for many important skills,[82] so to strengthen the trunk, a number of the activities in this section involve sitting up, reaching, and grasping.

Homemade Toy *Stacking Baby Blocks*

Soft blocks can be used for a fun developmental activity. Once your baby can grasp the blocks, he can bang them against the floor or each other, or you can stack them into a tower and your baby can swipe and knock them down. He will really get a kick out of this. As your little one's skills improve, he can even stack 2 or 3 blocks himself.

Here are simple instructions for making your own set of baby blocks. Collect a variety of different-sized milk cartons, small boxes, and toilet paper rolls. Be sure the cartons are washed and clean, then stuff each of the containers with newspaper or tissue paper. Be careful not to overstuff them. The boxes should not be rounded. Fold the ends down to create blocks and cylinders, then use masking or duct tape to close them securely. Use several different fun colors of contact paper or colorful duct tape to cover each block.

You now have a nice set of upcycled baby blocks!

Swings: Limit to 30 Minutes Daily

While many infants love the movement of a swing, others dislike the sensation. Gentle, rhythmic movement is good for your infant's developing sensory system, but swings can be overused. When baby's skull rests against the hard plastic shell, excess pressure is placed on his head, possibly leading to a flat spot. In addition, excess time in a swing can be stressful to a growing infant's spine because his legs hang down with all of his body weight supported by the bottom of his spine. If you have an infant swing, I recommend your baby spend no more than approximately 30 minutes each day in this piece of equipment and avoid using the swing for sleep. Fortunately, there are other options to incorporate rhythmic movement into his routine.

Activities That Address Posture and Balance

The following activities provide positive alternatives to the swing and help with the development of posture and balance:

Activity #1: Be My Baby

Position your infant tummy down on a blanket, sit down beside him, and use your leg like a bolster. Here's how: place your infant's arms over your thigh with his arms and hands reaching out in front. This provides support for his upper body while working his neck, back, and trunk muscles. It also strengthens his arm and hand muscles.

Once your infant is comfortable in this position, take his homemade rattle and hold it out in front of him. Shake it to coax him to focus on the rattle. Once he sees it, he'll likely reach for it with one hand. Tap on the toy if he doesn't seem interested in reaching for and grasping the rattle. Once he has it in his hand, guide him through shaking motions to show how the

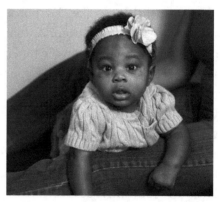

Be my baby

rattle makes noise. To help him understand that the rattle creates the sound, as he shakes it, say, "Wow! You're making a noise when you shake the rattle!" In this way you're teaching him about the concept of cause and effect.

Gently move the hand holding the rattle toward his empty hand and see if he will transfer the rattle from one hand to the other. If he doesn't do so on his own, give him a little help. By doing this, you're helping him learn how to use both hands together and encouraging crossing the body's midline—important precursors for lifelong skills such as walking, typing, catching a ball, reading, and writing.

Activity #2: Free Fallin'

When your infant is in a side-lying position, help him push up onto his elbow closest to the floor so that he's propping up on that elbow. You may need to place one of your hands just under his rib cage to help him prop himself up. From that position, help him sit upright.

Take the upcycled blocks and stack them in front of him. Encourage him to bat at and reach for them. Make sure the blocks are positioned closely enough in front of your infant so he can reach them easily. As you stack the blocks, be sure to explain what you are doing by saying things like, "I'm putting this blue block on the bottom. Watch! I'm placing the red block on the top." After the blocks are stacked, give your infant an opportunity to knock them over. If he doesn't attempt this on his own, guide his free hand in knocking

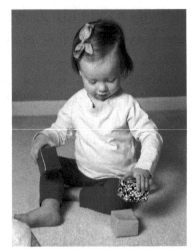

Free fallin'

them over. Most infants absolutely love to see and hear the blocks tumble to the ground! If your infant is tolerating the activity well, stack the blocks up again and repeat the activity with him in a propped position on his opposite side, or try it while he's sitting upright!

Activity #3: I'm Gonna Get You, Baby

To improve your infant's balance, sit him upright in your lap facing you. Hold him at the hips for support and say, "I'm going to get you," while leaning forward and kissing him on the cheek, neck, or tummy. Each time you say, "I'm going to get you," lean him slightly backward or slightly back and to one side. You can also slightly lift one of your legs, which will require him to shift his weight to stay in an upright position. Alternate lifting each leg while reciting "I Have a Little Bicycle" for a super-fun time. Your little one will love the interaction, and the adjustments he has to make as you play with him are great for his balance skills.

✿ ✿

I Have a Little Bicycle

I have a little bicycle
I ride it to and fro
And when I see the big green light
I know it's time to go

I have a little bicycle
I bought it at the shop
And when I see the big red light
I know it's time to stop

✿ ✿

Homemade Toy Squishy Sock Balls

Good old-fashioned balls that come in all sizes are great for infant play. Take several different sizes of clean, colorful socks and cut them to 1¼-inch in diameter or larger. Stuff each completely with cotton fiberfill. Cut several large squares from a soft package of baby wipes and place these inside the sock with the fiberfill so it makes a crinkly sound when squeezed. Securely stitch the open end of the sock closed. Your little one will enjoy the crinkly sound as he plays with the ball. Time to practice holding and throwing!

While he is sitting on your lap, if you notice your infant is having difficulty holding his back up straight, be sure to give him some support by placing your hands around his rib cage.

Activity #4: Getting Stronger Every Day

Take the large upcycled bolster pillow and position your infant over it lengthwise with his arms and legs straddling it in a crawling position. This allows him to bear weight on his hands and knees while having a little support. This is also a good position for him to reach for a toy such as his homemade rattle, using one hand while bearing weight on both knees and the other hand. Just hold and shake the rattle slightly in front of him, letting him reach for and grab it.

While your infant is still positioned this way, remove the bolster. His legs should already be tucked underneath his tummy with his knees bent in a crawling position. Place the rattle just out of reach in front of him, then position your forearm on the floor behind his feet, providing a surface he can push against.

You can even gently push against his feet to encourage him to return the pressure. He will enjoy pushing with his feet to propel himself slightly forward. Give him a bit of pressure on his bottom if he can't quite push off on his own. He'll feel motivated to get the toy in front of him.

Your goal? Give your infant plenty of opportunities to be successful while also encouraging movement and exploration. This activity improves his leg strength and is a precursor to crawling.

Activity #5: Having a Ball!

Once your infant is able to sit upright with a straight back, he's in a great position to play ball. While he's sitting, make sure to have soft blankets or a nursing pillow around him to prevent him from toppling over. Place your handmade ball or an 8- to 10-inch soft ball on the floor in front of him and roll it slowly back and forth. Show him how to push the ball away from himself using both hands, guiding him if needed the first time.

Now sit in front of and across from him several feet away. Slowly roll the ball to him so it lands where one of his hands can touch it. Encourage him to roll the ball back to you. As his rolling skills improve, you can scoot back a bit. This activity addresses your infant's sitting balance as well as his eye-hand coordination and bilateral skills.

If you notice your infant slumping with a rounded back, it means he's tired or not quite ready for independent sitting. If that's the case, sit on the floor and position him between your legs facing away from you so that he has your body to support his back. Sit close to a wall so that when he rolls the ball, it will bounce against the wall and come back to both of you.

Activity #6: Boot Scootin' Boogie

Position your infant on his stomach on a blanket and place the roly-poly toy that you made in Chapter 2 on one side of him, just out of reach to encourage him to pivot toward the toy. Be sure to position the roly-poly slightly to his front and side in his line of vision, motivating him to scoot toward it.

When your infant touches the toy with his hand, it should roll a bit. Watch him move toward the toy to make it roll again. Then tell him, "Good boy! You made the roly-poly move! Can you do it again?" After several pivots to one side, switch the toy to the opposite side. Alternating sides strengthens the muscles on both sides of his body. This wonderful pre-crawling activity strengthens his neck, arm, and trunk muscles.

Activity #7: Crossing the Line

Place your baby's homemade rattle in his right hand. After he plays with it for a minute, ask him to give it to you by encouraging him to cross his midline to place it in your outstretched hand. Shake the rattle several times and then place it in his left hand. Encourage him to "shake, shake, shake" the rattle, then prompt him to cross his midline in the opposite direction and give it to you. Now it's your turn to shake the rattle again!

Truth Be Told

One of your infant's favorite sounds is his mother's voice, so don't be shy—sing a lovely melody to your little one and watch the delighted response you receive. If you're not fond of your singing voice, then chat away. Your infant doesn't care, as long as he hears your voice!

If your infant hasn't started crawling by 7 months of age, he's probably rolling from front to back and back to front and sitting unsupported for several minutes. Once he begins to crawl on his hands and knees independently, take appropriate precautions. Because babies are naturally curious, provide plenty of protection, such as safety gates to confine him to safe areas and safety latches on all lower cabinets and drawers. Cover electrical outlets and keep the floors clean and clear. As you likely know, infants love to put *everything* in their mouths!

As you continue to spend quality time with your little one, the connection between the 2 of you grows. The precious time you are spending together helps him to continue to establish trust in you, as well as others. If your infant is playing independently for short periods, encourage this. When he shows an interest in toys, give him some space and allow him to play on his own at times. Watch for those small windows when he begins to entertain himself, acknowledge this bit of independence, and back off. This is the perfect opportunity for increasing your little one's attention span and encouraging independence. His attention span will gradually increase, and little by little he'll play on his own for longer periods.

Choosing a Child Care Center

Selecting a child care center can be a daunting task. You will likely visit several programs before making a final decision. Here are some questions to ask while you are there. Having the answers to these questions will help you make an informed choice that you feel comfortable with.

- Is the center licensed, registered, and/or accredited? Remember, it is perfectly fine to ask to see the appropriate supporting documentation.

- Has everyone who works at the facility had state and national background checks, including fingerprinting?
- Will you be allowed to visit your infant at any time if you call ahead? How are visitors screened?
- What is the adult to child ratio for each age group of children? *Note:* The American Academy of Pediatrics recommends no more than 3 infants younger than 12 months for each adult caregiver.
- Will your infant be supervised at all times, even when sleeping?
- Do the director and/or lead teachers have college degrees? If so, did they study child development or early childhood education?
- Does the program have a discipline policy that outlines how behavioral issues are handled? If so, does it state that spanking or excluding children is not allowed?
- Are the facility and classrooms clean, neat, and safe?
- Is a regular schedule followed that includes play, rest, and mealtimes?
- Is the setting warm and inviting, and are the teachers actively engaged with the babies?
- Have the adults in the program been trained on how to prevent child abuse and how to recognize and report signs of abuse?
- Have all the caregivers been trained in pediatric cardiopulmonary resuscitation (CPR), first aid, and how to prevent child abuse? Is there an emergency/disaster plan in place?
- What plan does the program follow if an infant is sick, injured, or lost?[83]

CHAPTER 8

Enhancing Development With Retro Activities: 7 to 9 Months

Between 7 and 9 months, your infant will amaze you with her rapid emotional and physical development. She will likely learn to sit, stand, and possibly even crawl during this period. This is a wonderful age for playing and interacting with your infant because around this time, she's also starting to gain more control over her hands and play more actively. Get ready to have fun!

Developmental Milestones: 7 to 9 Months

Look for your infant to display the following skills during this 7- to 9-month phase of growth:

- During tummy time, raises shoulders and shifts weight from side to side
- When lying on tummy, can pivot body in a circle
- Reaches and obtains toy
- Transfers toy from hand to hand
- Shakes rattle in imitation
- Pokes at toy with index finger
- Sits unsupported with a straight back
- Rakes toy with thumb and index fingers
- Holds a toy in one hand while reaching with the other
- Picks up food to place in mouth

Toy Tips: 7 to 9 Months

The following toys are appropriate for facilitating your infant's development during this age range. These items should never be left in the crib with your infant when she is sleeping.

- Soft stacking blocks
- Nesting blocks
- Soft books
- Board books
- Balls
- Musical toys
- Baby-safe photo album
- Push-pull toys
- Cause-and-effect toys
- Dolls
- Stuffed animals

Emerging Skill: Sitting Upright With Control

By the time your infant is developmentally ready to sit upright independently, she has gained a number of skills. Her head control is great, and her balance reactions are improving swiftly. If you hold her in a sitting position and gently tilt her to the side, forward, or backward, she will likely catch herself with one or both hands. As discussed in Chapter 7, when first learning to sit, your baby will prop herself up by placing both hands in front of her. As her balance improves and the muscles in her trunk get stronger, she will bring a hand to one side or another to keep her balance, and she will eventually sit upright without the use of either hand. She will be so proud of herself!

To support the development of balance and coordination, once your infant is able to sit up with a straight back independently, it's a good idea to let her play in this position as much as possible. With you by her side, she will learn to transition from her stomach to her hands and knees, then up to sitting. And don't forget to limit your infant's time in bouncers, carriers, and other baby gear.

Infant Temperament

You have probably noticed that your baby already has her own unique personality or temperament. From the early months after birth, all infants approach and react to the world around them in different ways. There are 3 styles of infant temperament and all have their strengths: easy or flexible, cautious or slow to warm up, and challenging or intense.[84] Infants with easy temperaments tend to have regular sleeping and eating habits and are generally happy and adaptable. Those who are cautious tend to be fearful of new situations and require time to warm up, while challenging or intense infants tend to react to their surroundings in a negative or extreme manner. Challenging infants typically do not have regular eating and sleeping habits and are sensitive to noises and other sensory stimulation. Of course, not all infants fit neatly into 1 of the 3 temperament styles; some are a mixture of the different styles. It is important to understand and appreciate your baby's unique personality, as different parenting approaches are often needed for infants with different temperaments. Some need more support, guidance, and reassurance, while others thrive by making their own way in the world. The amazing thing about your infant's temperament is that it forms the foundation of who she will be in the future!

Bumbo Baby Seat: Use Only With Supervision and Limit Use to 15 Minutes a Day

Guidelines that come with the Bumbo Baby Seat recommend it not be used with babies younger than 8 weeks due to safety concerns. Additionally, it should not be used on a raised surface, such as a countertop or kitchen table. Active babies can climb out of the molded plastic seat, fall, and become injured. Many babies have also been seriously hurt because they arched their backs, leaned, or rocked, causing the seat to tip over.

Because of serious injuries resulting from falls, including skull fractures, the US Consumer Product Safety Commission issued a voluntary recall of the Bumbo seat in August 2012. Consumers can contact the manufacturer to request a repair kit that includes a restraint belt with a warning label, installation and safe-use instructions, and a new warning sticker.[85] Always follow the safe-use instructions, and even when the Bumbo is used on the floor, provide constant supervision—no exceptions.

If you already have a Bumbo seat, your infant should be able to sit up well when using it. You should also limit your infant's time in it to no more than 15 minutes a day. Why? Because the seat holds a baby's hips in an unnatural position and fosters poor posture overall. Specifically, when in the Bumbo, your baby's hips tilt backward, causing her back to be rounded. Her hips essentially get "stuck" in one position, so when she reaches or rotates her trunk, she doesn't shift any weight. Not good. Instead, it's better to have your infant sit upright in the middle of a nursing pillow for support.

Activities to Build Balance and Strength

Help your infant gain strength and flexibility with the following activities. Many of these activities will still be appropriate when your infant passes the 9-month mark.

Activity #1: Sitting Pretty

Position your infant in front of you on the floor in a sitting position, facing away from you so you can place your hands on her hips for support as needed. Guide her forward so she's propped with both hands in front of her. Place your hands on top of hers, and guide her slightly back to an upright position, then forward again.

Once your infant can prop herself forward without guidance, you can help her improve her side-to-side balance. Select one of her favorite toys and position it slightly to her side and in front of her, making sure it's within her reach. Guide her in reaching for the toy with the hand opposite the toy, while she leans on the hand closest to the toy. When she grasps the toy successfully, praise her, switch the toy to the opposite side, and repeat the activity. Keep an eye on your infant's posture. If she starts to slump with a rounded back, it's time to take a break from this activity.

Activity #2: The Humpty Dance

Sit your infant upright on your lap. Gently bounce your legs up and down while softly singing a song or humming a tune. Your infant will be thrilled with the movement along with the melody! You can also position her tummy down and bounce her in this position. (Just don't do this if she has recently eaten!) Bouncing your infant like this is good for her balance and muscle control. You can even add a rocking chair to the mix! Rocking your infant provides another fun movement experience and is great for her sensory system.

Activity #3: Fly Me to the Moon

With your infant facing you, hold her by placing your hands around her rib cage, then slowly lift her up over your head and back down while saying, "Fly me to the moon!" Alternate lifting her up and down with moving her side to side. You can carry out this activity while you're seated or standing. Your infant will love it! If she seems fearful, however, move more slowly and talk to her in a calm, soothing voice as you lift her.

Activity #4: Every Day We Read the Book

Use your makeshift bolster or roll up a thin blanket to make a bolster, making sure it's firm enough to provide adequate support. Position your infant on her knees in front of the bolster with her bottom resting on top of both feet. Make sure her chest is in front of the bolster and position her arms over it. You'll find this to be a great position for your infant as you read to her. Position the personalized book just in front of her. This way, your infant can use her upper body muscles to push her hands against the floor, providing a good upper-extremity strengthening activity.

Give your little one guidance to turn each page of the book, taking the opportunity to teach concepts such as yes and no. For example, while looking at the pictures in the book, ask questions about what she sees. "Is this Mommy? Is this Daddy?" Be sure to allow plenty of time for her to respond through facial expressions, movements, or making noises. If she doesn't understand the question, help her by answering

Homemade Toy *My Very Own Book*

Have you noticed that it's difficult to find a simple picture book for babies these days? Books often have so many patterns or pictures on each page that it's difficult to teach your baby individual words or concepts without confusing her. This is why I always enjoyed making my own simple baby books, and my children loved them too!

I recommend using pictures from your everyday life, including your animals and close family members. Glue the pictures onto card stock; add a simple, creative story your baby will enjoy; and have the book laminated and spiral bound at a printing store. Or you can cover the pages with sticky-back laminate, hole-punch them, and put them in a binder, if you prefer. Another option is to use an old board book that no longer interests your baby. Cut card-stock paper so that it is the same size as the pages of the book (it is best if you trace a page to determine the exact size). After adding photographs and laminating the pages, glue each page onto the old board book. Make sure you put them in the correct order! Your baby will love having a personalized book!

yes or no and demonstrating it with an exaggerated nod or head shake. Watch to see if she vocalizes or tries to imitate you by moving her head. Be sure to use your words and happy expressions to encourage her attempts to copy you. If she's beginning to vocalize, encourage her to imitate "no." This activity provides a triple benefit: learning concepts as well as how to express herself verbally and nonverbally.

Activity #5: Balancing Act

You can help your infant develop her balancing skills with this fun activity. Once again, sit behind your infant, providing support by holding her just above her hips. Take one of her hands and move it to one side while shifting her weight to that same side. This will pull her slightly off balance. She should automatically place that hand on the floor for support. If she doesn't, give her a bit of guidance, moving her hand into the proper position. Be sure to practice this activity to her front and to the opposite direction. If she doesn't attempt to move her hand to hold herself up, she may not be ready for this activity. Wait several days and try again.

Activity #6: Rise and Shine

As your infant gains strength in her trunk and arms, it won't be long before she attempts to move from a side-lying position to sitting upright. A wonderful exercise is to guide her through the motions of this transition. When she's lying on her side, place your hand on the hip that she isn't lying on. Curl the fingers of your other hand around the side of her rib cage that's resting against the supporting surface. While guiding her trunk up with the hand holding her rib cage, guide her hips into a sitting position with your opposite hand at the same time. This activity should be repeated on the opposite side. As your infant gets stronger, she will require less guidance, and you can gradually reduce your assistance. The perfect opportunity to practice this activity is when changing a diaper or dressing your infant, because your little one will naturally be moving from side lying to sitting.

Activity #7: Tug-of-war

Hold one side of a blanket and place the other side in your baby's hands. Encourage her to hold on tight! Gently pull the blanket away from her and then give her an opportunity to pull it back. Alternate pulling and tugging with baby to strengthen her upper body.

Truth Be Told

It's a myth that babies don't have kneecaps. Actually, an infant's kneecaps are primarily made of soft cartilage to allow for the growth that takes place early in life. The kneecaps become much firmer throughout childhood as areas of bone form, and they continue to grow and increase in hardness throughout adolescence.[86]

Emerging Skill: Transferring Toys From One Hand to the Other

Now that your little one is reaching for and grasping items consistently, she'll begin to keep herself occupied for longer periods. She will enjoy picking up objects, examining and manipulating them, and she may even move objects from one hand to the other on her own. This significant accomplishment is a big boost to your infant's coordination skills. Provide as many opportunities to support this skill as possible by offering a variety of interesting, baby-safe items for your little one to manipulate and explore with her mouth.

Stationary Activity Center: Limit Use to 15 Minutes a Day

This piece of baby gear has a table with a sling-type seat that allows your baby to sit or stand, bounce, and rotate. When your baby is placed in an activity center, her legs are typically turned out from the hips, with her knees bent or extended. If her knees are extended, she usually stands on her toes, which is not good. While this position doesn't look comfortable, most babies don't seem to mind it and will play in an activity center for long periods without fussing, which is why you should limit your infant's time in this device to approximately 15 minutes a day. Unfortunately, the activity center doesn't encourage posture, body alignment, or movement patterns that are good for babies or advantageous for learning to walk. Because this is the developmental period for learning how to sit up, reach, and grasp, it's important to promote an upright posture and good body alignment.

If you have an activity center, it can come in handy once your infant begins to pull up into a standing position. Your little one can practice pulling up and standing outside the activity center to play with the toys. It basically becomes an activity table! Manipulating and playing with the toys from the outside of the activity center provides a boost for fine motor skill development.

A Variety of Fun Activities to Enhance Development

At this stage, your infant is learning fine motor coordination and enjoying sensory stimulation. Try these activities to expand her horizons.

Activity #1: Whole Lotta Stackin' Goin' On

Infants have lots of fun putting rings on a stacking ring toy and taking them off again; at this age, your infant may need assistance with putting the rings on the cone. Just place your little one in a seated position and sit behind her with your back supported against a wall or sofa. Pull her hips and back snugly against you so that your body provides support as needed. Another option is to place her seated upright in the center of a nursing pillow. Have your infant lean on one of her hands while reaching and grabbing for a ring with the other hand. Be sure to alternate the side on which you place each ring, and as she performs the actions, also incorporate language by saying, "You're putting the blue ring on the cone. Now

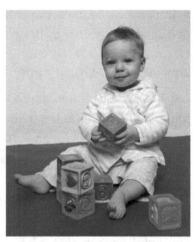

Whole lotta stackin' goin' on

you're taking the yellow ring off." This activity allows your infant to shift her balance to either side while bearing weight on each arm, shoulder, and hand, which is good for balance skills as well as hand development.

Your homemade blocks and colorful nesting containers are also great for stacking. Not only can you stack them, you can line them up by size, all while describing exactly what you are doing with your little one. "Look, Mommy is stacking the blocks one on top of the other. See how tall they are? Can you knock them down?" No doubt, knocking them down will be your infant's favorite part! After the blocks fall, place one of the smaller blocks in her hand and guide her in transferring it to her opposite hand, then back. This is a skill that will soon come naturally.

Activity #2: Hand It Over

Place a rattle or another fun toy in one of your little one's hands. Give her plenty of time to transfer the item to the opposite hand. After several minutes, if she hasn't switched the toy to the opposite hand, gently guide her empty hand toward the toy so it just touches the toy. Give her the opportunity to manipulate it with both hands. After several minutes, if she doesn't grasp the toy with her empty hand, place your hand over hers and help her close her fingers around it. You may need to encourage her to release the toy by rubbing the back of the grasping hand or distracting her with another toy. As this skill comes along, gradually decrease your assistance until your infant moves the items from one hand to the other by herself.

Activity #3: Happy Feet

Babies love to kick, and that is good because it strengthens their leg muscles and prepares them for walking. Put your infant on the floor lying on her back. Place an exercise ball at her feet and guide her in kicking the ball. (The exercise ball is perfect because it's large enough that your infant can see it move.) Once she understands that her foot is moving the ball, your infant will want to repeat the action over and over. Activities like this help your little one begin to understand the concept of cause and effect. Be sure to verbalize by saying, "Look! You made the ball move with your foot! What a big girl! Do you want to kick the ball again?" Look for a smile on her face that tells you she understands that her actions are causing the ball to move.

Activity #4: You've Got the Touch

A wide variety of sensory balls appropriate for baby play are available. These balls have various textured surfaces such as bumpy, smooth, slippery, and fuzzy. Let your little one hold and manipulate these balls during playtime for a rich sensory experience. Also, you can find a variety of textured items around the house (eg, blocks, toys, age-appropriate stuffed toys). While your infant is seated, place an empty plastic container in front of her. Demonstrate grasping the items and placing them into the container, then removing them. If she doesn't have good control with grasping and releasing yet, place your hand over hers and guide her through the motions. Be sure that any item you give her for play is large enough that choking is not a potential problem. If it can fit through a paper towel tube, it's too small.

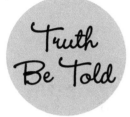

Your infant's sense of touch develops from head to toe. That's why she prefers to manipulate and examine items with her mouth.

Other than balls, developmentally appropriate toys with a variety of textures such as soft, firm, scratchy, and fluffy are available that will stimulate your infant's sensory system. Before she can grasp and release, place different toys in each hand for touch stimulation. Even at an early age, your baby will be able to discriminate differences in textures and enjoy the variety. Talk to your baby about the toys, explaining what they do, how they feel, and how they are different and alike. As she gets older, she will manipulate and explore the various qualities of each item.

Activity #5: Side Sitting

A great position to play with these tactile toys is side sitting. When your infant is sitting up with her legs straight out in front of her, move her legs slightly to one side and bend her knees. She should lean to the opposite side of her legs and prop on the opposite hand. Show her how to reach for toys in different directions using her free arm.

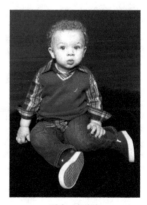

Side sitting

Activity #6: Reach for the Stars

When your infant is sitting up, sit in front of her. Hold a crinkle star to her right side near the floor and squeeze it to make it crinkle. Gently prompt her to reach for the star with her left hand. If she doesn't, give her a little guidance from her shoulder to reach for the shape. Her trunk

Homemade Toy *Crinkle Shapes*[87]

Babies absolutely adore these homemade crinkle shapes, and they aren't too difficult to make. Thanks to Joy's Hope (www.joyshope.com) for sharing the pattern!

You'll need the following supplies:

- Six ribbons.
- Flannel.
- Something crinkly like a wet-wipes package, but clear gift wrap or microwave popcorn wrappers are also nice and noisy.

Cut two 6-inch × 6-inch flannel squares and one 6-inch × 6-inch crinkle square. If you're an expert seamstress, try making different shapes, such as circles and stars. Cut six 4-inch pieces of ribbon.

Lay one flannel square right-side up. Pin folded ribbons along the edges with the folded edges turned inward. Place a second flannel square on top, right-side down. Pin all layers together with crinkle material on top.

Sew along all sides using a half-inch seam allowance. Be sure to leave enough room to turn it inside out. Take out all pins and trim excess ribbon, seams, and corners.

Turn it inside out. Tuck the raw edges in-between the ribbons. Topstitch around the entire square, making sure to close the opening.

Voilà!

should rotate slightly as she reaches across her midline for the item. Once she touches it, if she doesn't squeeze it, place your hand over hers and show her how to squeeze it and make it crinkle. Give her some time and see if she attempts to squeeze it on her own. Now hold your hand out to her left side and say, "Give me the star please." This is a great activity because the rotation keeps your infant's trunk flexible. You can also prompt her to transfer the star from hand to hand. She will enjoy the tactile sensation as well as the noise. Remember to alternate sides!

Activity #7: Find the Rattle

Take one of baby's rattles and shake it while it is out of her sight. It can be behind a blanket, under a table, or even in a shoebox. When she looks in the direction of the rattle, move it so she can see it. Hide the rattle again and reveal it so that it will appear in different places to encourage visual and auditory tracking.

Emerging Skill: Bearing Weight on Hands and Knees

It won't be long before your infant gains the strength to push up into a hands-and-knees position. During tummy time, you may notice her attempt to scoot across the room by pulling herself forward with her hands or bending and then extending her knees. She may even get up on her hands and knees and rock back and forth. Guess what? She's exercising those arm and leg muscles to prepare herself for crawling!

Baby Walkers: Avoid Use

Baby walkers have serious safety issues. Babies have fallen into pools, downstairs, and over ledges and been burned when using walkers, so don't take any chances—avoid this piece of equipment no matter what. In fact, because of safety issues, baby walkers are strongly discouraged by the American Medical Association, and they're no longer manufactured or sold in Canada.

Like baby gear we've discussed previously, baby walkers also promote undesirable positioning and poor alignment of baby's back. Physical therapists suggest that walkers actually delay, not help, a baby in learning to walk. Babies who use walkers tend to crawl less, and the large trays prevent them from naturally exploring and manipulating nearby objects, which is important for cognitive development.[88] Taking all of these factors into consideration, it's best to "just say no" to baby walkers![89]

Activities to Increase Strength and Develop Concepts and Language

Following are a variety of activities that support your infant's continued development:

Activity #1: Got Strength?

Position your infant on her hands and knees in front of you. Help her maintain this position by placing one of your hands just under her arm around her rib cage and the other just above the opposite hip. If she's getting close to staying in the position on her own, you can just give her some support by placing one hand on her hip and your other hand on her opposite elbow or by placing both of your hands on her hips. Her knees should be directly aligned under each hip, and each hand should be under the same shoulder. Talk to her the entire time, encouraging her to stay in the position for several seconds.

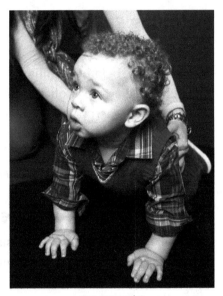

Got strength?

As she gains strength, provide guidance by gently rocking her backward, then forward. When you notice she doesn't need as much assistance, gradually provide less support.

Activity #2: See You Later, Alligator

Your infant is at the age where she's beginning to understand the concept of cause and effect. This is the perfect time to play a fun game of hide-and-seek with a rattle or stuffed animal. When she's seated upright in front of you, hide the item under a blanket or behind your back. If you're using the rattle, shake it while you are hiding it so she is watching you the entire time. If she loses interest once it's hidden, reveal part of the item and ask, "Where is the toy?" Give her a chance to reach for it and retrieve it while you say, "Oh! There it is!" Repeat the activity. At some point, you will no longer have to reveal part of the toy.

Activity #3: Talk to Me, Baby

Take advantage of playtime as an opportunity to model language for your infant. Express yourself through movement and gestures and speak to your baby in full sentences. Make sure what you say has meaning because your infant is always listening and learning! The "point and name" game is wonderful for your baby's language skills. Point to different objects or various body parts and name them, using complete sentences. For example, "Look, here is your nose"; "Wow, there is your elbow"; or "This is a red rattle!" Encourage your infant to point or touch what you are naming. This will help her understand that there is a connection between the words and objects or body parts.

Use different tones of voice while playing with your infant. For example, in a soft voice, tell her, "Listen, Mommy is whispering." Chatter away while spending time with her, telling your little one details about your day, such as what you did, where you went, or whom you saw. The more language, the better.

Activity #4: All in the Family

Take several photographs of family members and have them laminated. Show them to your little one during play, asking questions such as, "Is this your sister?" or "Is this Daddy?" Help her understand the concepts of yes and no by modeling the answers for her, nodding or shaking your head in an exaggerated manner as you do so. Introduce new concepts like, "Look, Mommy is a girl," or "See, Daddy is big and tall!"

Showing your infant pictures of family members and familiar objects helps develop recognition skills. Point to body parts and tell her, "This is Daddy's nose," and "Look at Mommy's hair." Infants love to look at faces and themselves at this stage, so use a baby mirror and point to her eyes, nose, mouth, and other features while explaining what she is seeing. For example, "Look! Baby is opening her mouth," or "Mommy is touching baby's nose."

Activity #5: If the Hat Fits...

You will need a colorful hat for this activity. When your infant is in a sitting position, sit just in front of her, place the hat on your head, and tell her, "Look! The hat is *on* my head." Then remove it and say, "Now the hat is *off*." Next, put the hat on and off your infant's head! Encourage her to reach for the hat and knock it off her head or your head while you model the term "off" in an exaggerated tone. Guide her hands through the motions of removing the hat the first time around if necessary.

Truth Be Told

You can use various toys to teach the concept of cause and effect. One way to introduce this skill is by showing your infant how you can roll one ball into another to make the second ball move. I always called this activity "bump the ball"! Pop-up and jack-in-the-box toys are also great for reinforcing this concept. When your infant pushes a button, something pops up. How cool is that?

Activity #6: Look at You, Baby!

Position a nonbreakable mirror in front of your infant so she can see her own reflection. Although she won't realize she's looking at herself yet, she'll feel delighted. Say, "Look, there's baby!" (Or use her name.) Talk about the reflection, describing and pointing to various facial features such as her nose, mouth, and eyes. Then say, "See? There is baby's nose. Mommy is touching your nose. Look at your ears. They are on either side of your head." Touch each body part as you say it so your little one will learn to recognize her body parts. While she's in this position, sing your baby a song. Babies love the classic tune, "You Are My Sunshine."

Activity #7: Hide and See

While your baby is positioned in front of the mirror looking at her reflection, cover her head with a very small baby blanket. Say, "Where did the baby go?" Then remove the small blanket so that she can see herself again. Say, "There she is!" Repeat the activity several times!

The Importance of Stress Management for Parents

Having a young baby can be a stressful experience, and even though stress is hard on parents, it is even harder on baby. Why? When an individual is stressed, this causes the fight-or-flight response. This is desirable if you are in a dangerous situation. For example, if you are out jogging and a rabid dog starts to chase you, cortisol and adrenaline are released into your system, causing your breathing to speed up and your heart to beat faster, sending extra blood to the muscles. This gives you a sudden burst of energy, allowing you to (hopefully!) flee to safety. But unfortunately, stress is contagious. Research tells us that infants can sense when their parents experience anxiety. Also, when parents are stressed out, they tend to engage less with their infant and be less responsive. This, in turn, causes the baby's cortisol and adrenaline levels to rise. Prolonged stress exposure in infancy can negatively influence brain development, leading to issues with memory, attention, and emotional control in the future. For this reason, it is important to be aware of your stress levels and how you react to stress so that it doesn't negatively affect your baby. On the other hand, being responsive to and physically affectionate with your baby will lower her stress levels and help her feel safe and secure.[90]

As your infant continues to develop physically and cognitively, she will begin to venture out and explore the environment. As a safety net, she will balance her exploration by frequently returning to you. Interestingly, research suggests that the quality of an infant's attachment to the primary caregiver directly affects how far and how often the infant will move away from the caregiver to explore and investigate her surroundings.[91] An infant who is securely attached to her parent will have the confidence to venture out and about, whereas an infant who is not securely attached will not leave her parent's side to explore the environment. As exposure and interaction with the environment directly influence brain development, your bond with your infant is very important for her future.

CHAPTER 9

Enhancing Development With Retro Activities: 10 to 12 Months

A re you ready to get busy? Life as you know it is about to change—
because if your infant isn't already mobile, he's about to be! Your
little one is at the brink of toddlerhood, which is a time full of excitement, energy, and exploration. From crawling, to pulling up, to cruising,
to walking independently, your child will stun you with how quickly he
masters these skills. This chapter contains a variety of fun and engaging movement experiences that will enrich your infant's development. If
you follow through with the activities in this section, you will spend lots
of quality time with your infant. And if you show all of your family members and your infant's caregivers how to carry out these activities, they
can have fun with your little one as well. It's a busy time, and it passes
quickly. So take a deep breath, keep reading, and get ready to have a
blast with your infant! Keep in mind that many of these activities will
still be appropriate for your baby when he's a little older.

Developmental Milestones: 10 to 12 Months

Look for your infant to display the following skills during this 10- to
12-month phase of growth:
- Bears weight on hands and knees and rocks back and forth
- Crawls several feet on hands and knees
- Gets into sitting position independently
- Points with index finger
- Can easily release objects

- Catches self with hands if thrown off balance while seated
- Attempts to imitate a scribble after seeing a demonstration
- Imitates sounds
- Tries to say at least 1 word
- Removes lid from box
- Bangs toys together in play
- Places 1 cube or block in a cup
- Drops a toy deliberately
- Removes cover to obtain hidden toy
- Brings spoon from bowl to mouth
- Points
- Waves goodbye
- Imitates actions
- Pulls to stand
- Stands alone
- Plays patty-cake
- Cruises while holding onto furniture

Toy Tips: 10 to 12 Months

The following toys are appropriate for facilitating your infant's development during this age range. Never leave these toys in the crib with your infant when he is sleeping.

- Shape sorter
- Stacking rings
- Soft stacking blocks
- Cloth books
- Plastic mirror
- Toy telephone
- Toy dolls/stuffed animals
- Pounding bench
- Connectable beads
- Toys that "say" words
- Toy drum

Emerging Skill: Pulling to Stand

Crawling on his hands and knees has made your infant much stronger, and strong arms and legs make it easier for him to pull himself up and stand. Because he's naturally curious and interested in exploring his surroundings, standing is the perfect opportunity to discover the many goodies that have been out of his reach all this time. Standing while holding your hands or onto a piece of furniture strengthens his legs and ankles and helps him develop the balance he needs to stand on his own.

Smart Toys: Limit Use

Earlier in the book, we discussed how smart toys incorporate computer technology that allows the toys to respond to an infant's actions in some way or another. Many of these toys can even recognize an infant's skill level and respond appropriately. Some smart toys are supposed to teach letters, numbers, and words, but your infant just passively observes once the toy is activated. No further interaction or engagement takes place. In one research study, when babies and parents played together with smart toys, the parents used fewer words, initiated conversation less, and responded to their infants fewer times than those who played with traditional toys. Also, the babies who played with the smart toys vocalized less.[92] On the other hand, dress-up clothes, puzzles, stacking rings, and blocks all facilitate development and promote active play. Compared with smart toys, which tend to entertain, I would opt for interactive toys any day. (In general, it's best to select toys that don't require batteries.) Let's go retro and encourage old-fashioned play and creativity!

Activities for Strength, Balance, and Vision

The following activities will support your infant's strength, balance, and visual tracking:

Activity #1: I'm Still Standing

This is a fun activity to carry out once your infant is strong enough to stand with support. Grasp your infant's hands while he's sitting on the floor. Raise your arms slowly, lifting him up to a standing position. Once he's up, let him stand for 8 to 10 seconds and look at his surroundings, then slowly lower him back into a sitting position. This is a great way to strengthen the muscles in his arms, legs, and bottom. Of course, it's always more fun if you incorporate a song or rhyme! Use one like "The Grand Old Duke of York," or make up your own!

❖ ❖

The Grand Old Duke of York

The grand old Duke of York
He had 10,000 men
He marched them up to the top of the hill
Then he marched them down again.
And when they were up, they were up
And when they were down, they were down
And when they were only halfway up
they were neither up nor down.

❖ ❖

Activity #2: Bebop Baby

This is another great activity for balance. While facing your infant with him seated upright on the floor, separate his legs just enough to place a medium-sized ball directly in front of him. Show him how to roll the ball in your direction, then roll the ball back to him. This is a fun and engaging activity, and it's great for teaching the concept of turn taking. When your little one has the ball, tell him, "It's your turn to roll the ball.

Good boy! You rolled the ball! Now it's Mommy's turn to roll the ball. Get ready, the ball is coming back to you."

Roll the ball to his right side on the outside of his leg so that he has to rotate his trunk to retrieve the ball. After he rolls it back to you, roll the ball to his left side. The rotation is good for his flexibility and balance.

Activity #3: At the Hop

Time to pull out the exercise ball again! Sit your infant upright on the ball, holding him at his hips. Roll the ball slowly back and forth. Once he's accustomed to the motion, while still holding him, push your infant's bottom downward, then back up, providing a gentle bouncing motion. If he seems fearful, you may be bouncing too hard, and you'll need to ease up. You can even slowly alternate rocking and bouncing the ball. Always keep both of your hands on your infant the entire time to keep him safe. Most likely, your little one will smile from ear to ear during this activity.

Activity #4: Toss-up

Another option is to bounce your infant on your knee and toss him gently into the air. Use moderation with these activities, as you don't want to overstimulate him. Also be aware of his facial expressions and stop if he isn't enjoying it. Share a traditional rhyme like "A Bouncing We Will Go" with your infant as you bounce him.

❋ ❋

A Bouncing We Will Go

A bouncing we will go

A bouncing we will go

High ho the derry-o

A bouncing we will go.

❋ ❋

Homemade Toy *Put a Ring on It*

Your baby will find this simple homemade toy totally entertaining. All you need is a plastic baby spoon and a variety of rings (eg, shower curtain rings, plastic curtain rings, teething rings). Show your baby how to hold the handle of the spoon with one hand and place the rings on the other end of the spoon with the other. This wonderful activity encourages motor planning and requires both hands to work together.

Activity #5: Marching On

To exercise your infant's trunk and hip muscles, hold him in a standing position with his feet on your thighs while you're seated on a chair, couch, or ottoman. He can face toward or away from you. Hold him at his hips and slowly alternate moving each of your legs up and down so he is making stepping motions. If he's facing you and supporting himself with ease while standing, just hold his hands during this exercise. Your infant will enjoy this activity even more if you sing a marching song as you're taking him through the motions.

When the Saints Go Marching In

Oh, when the saints go marching in

Oh, when the saints go marching in

Oh, how I want to be in that number

When the saints go marching in!

Activity #6: Stand and Play

Sit on the floor beside a sofa, an ottoman, or a low chair and help your infant into a standing position in front of the chair or sofa. Bring his arms in front of him and position them on the seat of the chair or sofa so that he can use them for occasional support. The homemade "put a ring on it" toy should be within his reach. If needed, place one of your hands on your infant's tummy and one on his bottom for support. Be sure that he is in a nice position, with his head, shoulders, hips, and knees all aligned. Encourage him to play with his ring toy while you provide standing support as needed. Don't forget to praise him when he successfully places a ring on a spoon! If he doesn't attempt to stand up with your support, that means he's not ready for this activity. Just wait and try it again when he's a little older.

Activity #7: Barefoot Baby

Don't be in a rush to put shoes on your baby. When your infant goes barefoot, it allows him to feel the surface on which he is standing and adjust his balance as needed. Additionally, research has found that wearing shoes can affect a child's gait by reducing foot motion.[93] So ditch the shoes when you can and bring on those bare feet!

Truth Be Told

Research reveals that it's possible to foster creativity in our little ones, especially when they're young.[94,95] Creativity is basically a way of solving problems. However, it's different in that it involves solving problems for which there's no easy answer—so the problem solver has to be adaptable, flexible, and original. As parents, we can foster creativity in our children by offering an environment that encourages free play and exploration. Be sure to expose your child to a stimulating environment with as much reading, music, and movement as possible.

Emerging Skill: Standing Independently

A major prerequisite to walking is the ability to stand independently. The best way to prepare your infant for standing is to provide plenty of floor time and encourage crawling. To help your infant learn how to stand on his own, catch him while he's standing and holding on to a piece of furniture (something soft like a sofa—no sharp edges!). Sit about 2 feet away from him, hold one of his favorite toys close to the hand that he's using to support himself, and see if he'll reach for the toy. Be patient and don't rush him. He may start to reach, then hold on again for support, which is fine. He's developing his balancing skills. Over time, he will gain the strength and balance needed to reach for and grasp the toy without holding on.

Jumping Devices: Avoid Use

These products have a variety of names, including Johnny Jump Up, Jumperoo, and Jump & Go. Some attach to doorframes, while others are freestanding, similar to a stationary activity center. Although it's likely your baby would enjoy one of these products, they present potential risks. A device that suspends from a doorframe poses dangers such as head trauma, strangulation, and whiplash. All of the jumpers encourage standing on the tiptoes, which is not good for baby's feet, and excess jumping in these devices puts unnecessary stress on your infant's legs, hips, and spine. Considering the negative effect these products have on infant development, they're not worth the risk.

More Activities to Enrich Experience

The following activities cover balance, music, colors, shapes, and body awareness:

Activity #1: Rock on, Baby!

Once your infant is able to stand without help, you can help him with his balance by carrying out this activity. Sit behind or in front of him and hold him at his hips. Slowly shift his body weight from one leg to the other in a side-to-side rocking motion, making sure his arms are free so he can use them for balancing. This activity is extra fun if you incorporate a nursery rhyme such as "Hickory Dickory Dock."

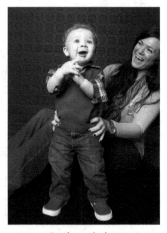

Rock on, baby!

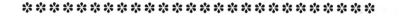

Hickory Dickory Dock

Hickory, dickory, dock,

The mouse ran up the clock.

The clock struck one,

The mouse ran down,

Hickory, dickory, dock.

Activity #2: Hide-and-seek Time

For visual stimulation during play, use toys with black-and-white contrast. You might use a stuffed animal such as a zebra or a panda and play hide-and-seek by placing the item behind your back and asking, "Where is the panda?" Give your infant plenty of time to look for the panda, but if he doesn't, revealing a panda arm or leg should do the trick.

If you have a squeeze toy that squeaks, show it to your infant, then hide it behind your back or under a blanket. Ask him, "Where did the toy go?" and then squeeze it. Make it squeak several times, giving your little one plenty of time to look for the toy, before you reveal the hiding place. Remember to speak slowly, clearly, and in complete sentences during play.

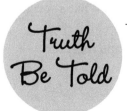

The relationship between music and language plays a role in an infant's language development, as music fosters communication skills.[96]

Activity #3: Play It Again, Please

If you play a musical instrument, this is the perfect way to entertain your infant. You can play music and sing, and I assure you, your child will be fascinated. If you don't play an instrument, you can purchase a toy xylophone and play it for him. It's simple. Just follow the instructions! Once you have demonstrated how to tap on the keys, let your infant make music using the xylophone as well. It's a wonderful, engaging way to introduce rhythm and music to your child!

Homemade Toy Baby Drums

Almost every adult remembers making a drum as a child. It's as easy as covering an oatmeal box or coffee can with colorful contact paper and using 1 or 2 plastic baby spoons as drumsticks. Of course, you can always give your child a saucepan and a short wooden spoon. Playing with objects from the kitchen cabinets has never been so much fun!

Activity #4: Beat It

Using your new homemade drum, show your infant how to tap the drum using the palms of your hands, then give him a chance to imitate you. Once he has that down pat, demonstrate tapping the drums using your fingertips. Give him time to master that skill. Finally, show him how to beat the drums using the plastic baby spoons. Have him hold the handles of each spoon in the palms of his hands and tap-tap-tap away. Sing a song while he plays the drums. He's working on motor skills and coordination while he's experiencing music and rhythm. If you made 2 drums, play alongside your infant; if you want to thoroughly entertain him, occasionally imitate the drum patterns he makes. What a special way to get to encourage an early love of music in your child!

Here is a fun song to sing as you and your baby drum together.

✽✽✽✽✽✽✽✽✽✽✽✽✽✽✽✽✽✽✽✽✽✽✽✽✽✽

Skidamarink

Skidamarink a-dink a-dink,

Skidamarink a-doo,

I love you.

Skidamarink a-dink a-dink,

Skidamarink a-doo,

I love you.

I love you in the morning

And in the afternoon;

I love you in the evening

And underneath the moon.

Oh, skidamarink a-dink a-dink,

Skidamarink a-doo,

I love you!

✽✽✽✽✽✽✽✽✽✽✽✽✽✽✽✽✽✽✽✽✽✽✽✽✽✽

Truth Be Told

As you know from reading Chapter 2, sucking is a reflex, and it is actually one of the most common reflexes seen during infancy. Babies often suck on their thumbs, fingers, or a pacifier to help them feel secure and relaxed during the first 12 to 24 months after birth. So don't be concerned about thumb-, finger-, or pacifier sucking at this early age because your infant will likely grow out of it. If the habit is still present when your child's adult teeth start to come in, speak with your child's pediatrician.

Activity #5: Get Smart

Take advantage of every opportunity you can to teach your infant new concepts as you play together. Reading a book about a particular concept such as shapes, for example, is one fun way to teach your infant about that concept. Now that he is older, be sure to encourage your infant to turn the pages of the book by himself. Shape-sorting toys are also a great option because he can actually manipulate the shapes as you explain details such as, "A square has 4 corners," and "A circle is round and smooth."

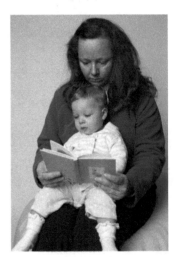

Get smart

Playing actively with simple toys is a wonderful opportunity to familiarize your infant with different concepts. During play, you can use different toys to demonstrate and explain to him the concepts of beside, between, on top of, under, in front of, and behind. For example, you can position 2 stuffed animals on the floor in front of your infant and take another stuffed animal and alternate its position, saying, "Look! Teddy bear is under the table, and now he is sitting *on top of* the table." Use your imagination, making teddy bear dance and act silly.

You can also work on skills of categorizing with your infant by grouping similar items by size. Create 2 piles of toys, the big toys pile and the small toys pile, and tell him which toys go best in which pile. Your infant will have fun with these activities and learn new concepts all the while.

Introducing the concepts of *same* and *different* is a fun activity. You can show your infant stuffed animals and put all the dogs together, saying, "These are the same. They are all dogs." You can even introduce the concepts by categorizing toys by color, shape, and size.

Activity #6: Hokey Pokey

I'm sure you remember the "Hokey Pokey" song. Of course you do! The hokey pokey is a great activity to help your infant increase body awareness. Sit him upright in your lap and sing the "Hokey Pokey" song while taking turns holding each of his extremities and moving it gently around. You remember how it goes: "You put your right hand in, you put your right hand out, you put your right hand in, and you shake it all about!" Your infant will get the giggles when you "shake it all about."

Activity #7: Feely Feet

When your baby is barefoot, give him opportunities to stand or walk on a variety of different surfaces, such as carpet, linoleum, and grass. Talk to him and describe the way the surfaces feel as he is experiencing them.

Emerging Skill: Cruises or Walks With or Without Support

As your infant's gross motor skills continue to develop, he has more opportunities to get mobile and interact with his surroundings. Once he is standing up with good strength and balance, the next big accomplishment is cruising along furniture. Basically, your infant holds on to a sofa or chair for support and sidesteps to get where he wants to go. This is great because as he steps to the side, he's learning how to shift his weight and keep his balance, which is a skill that he will use for walking. For safety's sake, be sure that whatever your infant holds while cruising does not have sharp edges and is secure enough to support him as he moves along. This is a precursor to walking, so get ready—it won't be long before he's toddling all over the place!

Walking Harnesses: Limit Use

Walking harnesses have a number of different names, including walking assistant and harness walk. Basically, the product is designed to help an infant learn how to walk. It has a harness or vest that fastens around an infant's chest, with adjustable straps attached to the back of the harness for parents to hold while the infant is walking. This product is supposed to help an infant learn to walk and balance more naturally, with less hands-on assistance from parents, limiting falls for him and fewer backaches for parents from bending over. In theory this sounds great, but it's important not to rush your infant into walking by using a walking harness before he's ready. If your little one doesn't have the postural control and balance needed for walking and you push him before he's ready, this could make him fearful, which is a major no-no. I have also heard parents complain that the harness rides up and cuts off the circulation under their infant's armpits or that their infant leaned forward while using it. The bottom line: as parents, we should never rush our child's development, only support him when he's ready.

Keep Your Infant Safe: Secure the Area

Now that your infant is mobile, it won't be long before the climbing begins. That means it's time to remove any large or heavy items from tables, shelves, and dressers. Most importantly, secure any furniture that might tip over if your infant pulls up on it or attempts to climb it. There are numerous safety straps and brackets designed to anchor furniture such as tall lamps, televisions, television stands, bookshelves, dressers, and chests to the wall that will keep your precious little one safe. It is also important to use cordless products if possible; if the blinds or curtains have cords, make sure there are no loops and that cord stops are installed to prevent the formation of a loop.

Activities to Expand Horizons

The following activities support cruising and walking, help your little one enjoy the outdoors and sensory experiences, and develop language and muscle coordination:

Activity #1: Look Who's Cruising

If your infant seems interested in cruising, you can give him a little assistance that will help him gain the strength and coordination needed for this skill. While he is standing at a sofa or soft chair, place his favorite toy just out of his reach to one side. If he doesn't attempt to move toward it, place your hand just above one hip and shift his weight onto the leg on the opposite side of the toy. This will cause him to lift the leg closest to the toy so he can sidestep toward it. Once he lifts that leg, provide guidance with your hands, gradually moving the lifted leg toward the toy, allowing him to take the step. His opposite leg should follow, and you can give it a little help if needed. Always repeat the activity to the other side so that both sides of his body get stronger.

Activity #2: Moving on Up

While sitting behind your infant, help him kneel in front of an ottoman, a sofa, or a low chair so his elbows and hands are resting on the seat surface. Make sure his body and legs are aligned with each other and he's holding his head up straight. This position strengthens muscles in the legs, hips, and trunk, which improves posture. Place your hands on his hips and press down gently on his right hip, shifting his weight onto his right leg. Carefully lift his left leg and bend his knee, bringing him into a

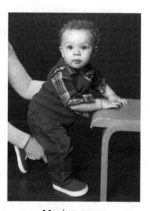

Moving on up

half-kneeling position. From this position, he's halfway to standing. Let him try to pull up the rest of the way on his own, only giving him help if he needs it. Wow! Your infant is getting so strong!

Homemade Bubbles

Blowing bubbles is a blast, and it's a great activity indoors or out-doors. It encourages visual tracking, and your infant will be thor-oughly entertained watching bubbles float and pop. You can also model popping bubbles using your index finger. If your infant doesn't imitate you, give him hand-over-hand guidance so he can pop them. This is a real treat, and it's great for teaching him how to isolate his index finger for pointing. You may want to save some money while having fun and make your own bubbles!

Mix the following ingredients together in a container:
- One-fourth cup baby shampoo
- Three-fourths cup water
- Three tablespoons corn syrup

Make the recipe an hour or two ahead of playtime for the very best bubbles.

Activity #3: Here Comes the Sun

Playtime shouldn't be limited to indoor activity. Nature provides a vast array of visual stimulation. Spread a soft blanket on a smooth, firm surface and enjoy time together in the great outdoors. You can go to a park or simply find the perfect spot in your own yard. Stay seated next to your infant for safety reasons and from there, point out interesting items in the environment such as birds, grass, and trees. Be sure to pro-tect your infant from the sun and consult with your child's pediatrician about the use of sunscreen once your little one reaches 6 months of age.

During outdoor tummy time, it's fun to have your infant look for vari-ous items in the environment. Ask him questions such as, "Do you see the brown dog?" Then point at the dog. Or "Can you find a big, green shrub?" This activity encourages visual exploration while keeping him entertained. You can also tell your infant to listen for different sounds. For example, "Did you hear the car drive by?" or "Listen. Daddy hears a train. Do you hear it?" And you could even look in that direction and cup your ear to give him a clue.

Don't forget to incorporate the sense of touch. Give your infant the opportunity to touch, hold, and feel items in the great outdoors, such as grass, leaves, and flowers. Just be cautious and don't let him put any of these items in his mouth!

Activity #4: Bye-bye, Baby

All that is needed for this activity are several stuffed animals and dolls. If your infant needs to improve his standing balance, have him stand against a wall. His back and bottom should barely touch the wall, and his hips, knees, and feet should all be aligned directly under his trunk. Standing close to the wall provides security and support for your little one. Kneel several feet in front of him. Hold one of the stuffed animals directly in front of him and tell him, "Say bye-bye to the bear." As you say this, wave the bear's hand to provide an example, and if necessary, wave your hand. If your infant doesn't understand, reach forward, guide his hand through the waving motions, then praise him. "Good job! You waved bye-bye to the bear!" Take the bear and put it out of sight.

Once again, kneel several feet in front of your infant. Take one of the dolls, hold it out to your far right, and say, "Wave bye-bye to dolly!" while moving one of the doll's hands up and down. Your infant will probably bring his hand over and wave it in the direction that you are holding the doll. If he doesn't understand, follow the same routine as before. It won't be long before your infant is waving bye-bye spontaneously; in the meantime, you have been working on standing balance and weight shifting. Way to go!

Activity #5: You Light Up My Life

Here's a fun activity to carry out before a bedtime story. Turn off or dim the light in the room and shine a penlight, flashlight, or light-up toy on the wall. Once your infant sees the light, move it slowly from one side of the room to the other and up and down to encourage visual tracking. Shine the light on various objects in the room. "Do you see the picture on the wall? Is that your stuffed animal?" You can also turn the light on and off, telling him, "Look! The light is on...and now it's off!" Shine the light on an object such as a chair. Say, "Look, there's a chair." Then turn off the light. "Where is the chair? Where did it go?" Turn the light back on, shining it on the chair, and say, "There it is!" This will surely bring about some giggles.

This activity is great for your infant's vision as he works on following the light with his eyes and focusing on the various objects you point out. If you shine the light on an object and turn the light off and on again, you are teaching your child the concept of object permanence.

Truth Be Told   Separation anxiety is a developmental stage that many infants begin to experience around 7 to 8 months of age. Some infants experience more intense separation anxiety than others. This depends on the infant's temperament and the setting. Certain infants react to a caregiver's absence with intense screaming and crying; others will respond very strongly and heatedly to caregiver absence by crying and fussing; others will look concerned and look around for a parent; and still others respond by only whimpering and whining.

Activity #6: Ain't No Pillow High Enough

Form a bunch of pillows and cushions into the shape of a nest and place your infant in the center. Make sure the pillows and cushions are large and stable. Provide support at your infant's hips if needed and help him climb up and over the pillows to get to the other side. He will be so proud of his accomplishment!

Toward the end of the first year, as your infant gains experience with mobility, his depth perception continues to develop, which means he will be able to better judge how far objects are away from him, as well as how far apart they are from one another. Also, as his attention span increases, your infant will show more interest in simple picture books. Looking at books provides the perfect opportunity to help him develop a love of books and reading. This is highly beneficial because there's strong evidence that reading with your child promotes brain development, improves future reading skills, and leads to future success in school.[97,98]

Activity #7: I Got a Feeling!

Show your baby a photo of you smiling or laughing. Ask him, "Is Mommy happy?" Encourage him to nod and say yes. You can also snap a photo of your baby when he is upset, show it to him later, and ask, "Were you sad when Mommy took this photo?" Then tell him, "Yes, you were sad." Then remind him, "But you are happy now!"

Social and Emotional Development

Early social and emotional development are very much interrelated.[99] For example, when an infant begins to recognize and identify his own feelings, he will be able to start understanding what others are feeling during social interactions. There are a variety of ways to nurture your infant's social and emotional development. Here are several!

- Make sure that your little one feels loved, safe, and secure. This allows him to bond with you, which is the foundation of social and emotional development.
- When you stick to a routine, such as a regular napping and feeding schedule, your baby will have an idea of what to expect throughout the day. This will also help him feel safe and secure.
- Take advantage of opportunities to identify the emotions your baby is experiencing and talk about the many different feelings that we all experience.
- Maintaining a regular sleep schedule plays an important role in healthy social-emotional development.[100]

As you've discovered, there are a vast array of opportunities for supporting all areas of your baby's development throughout the day. Remember, the more you talk to your little one, the richer his vocabulary will be. It's also important to say your infant's name frequently, as infants tend to listen better after they've heard their names. Continue to be enthusiastic about your infant's development, and you and your infant will both reap the rewards!

CHAPTER 10

Enhancing Development With Retro Activities: 13 to 24 Months

Your child's body and brain will make an amazing transformation between the ages of 13 and 24 months. She will astonish you as she continues to grow physically and develop her unique little personality. During this time, she becomes aware of your emotional expressions, and because she is making the connection that facial expressions are connected to internal feelings, she understands when you're upset or distressed.

As she enters her toddler years, she'll stay busy exploring the world around her as she interacts with her environment. In these months, watch her progress from walking to running, then on to jumping and climbing. Prepare yourself for some action!

Developmental Milestones: 13 to 24 Months

Look for your child to display the following skills during this phase of growth:

Thirteen to 18 Months

- Walks with or without support
- Squats down and picks up a toy
- Eats with fingers
- Turns pages of a board book
- Drinks from a cup independently

- Throws a ball underhand
- Stacks 4 blocks
- Removes basic clothing

Nineteen to 24 Months

- Runs with stiff legs
- Eats with spoon (some spillage)
- Kicks a ball forward with one foot
- Spontaneous scribbles
- Jumps in place 2 times
- Points to specific images in a book and points to named body parts

Activities: 13 to 24 Months

Activity #1: The Big Squeeze

At bath time, give your child a variety of sponges to play with. It's easy to take several colorful kitchen sponges and cut them into fun sizes and shapes to fit into your child's hand at bath time. A large square, small triangle, blue star, and green circle are all possibilities. Have fun and use your imagination! Show your little one how to sink a sponge underwater, watch it fill up, then hold it up and squeeze the water out. Not only will your little one enjoy this activity; she'll strengthen the tiny muscles in her hands as she plays.

Activity #2: Getting Down to Earth

You can help your child gain the strength needed for squatting by encouraging her to squat from standing. Hold an appealing toy just below her knees so she'll reach down for the toy. Once she begins to reach for it and bend her knees, move the toy closer to the floor. That way, she has to move deeper into a squatting position. Continue until you place the toy on the floor and she retrieves it.

Activity #3: Shop 'Til You Drop

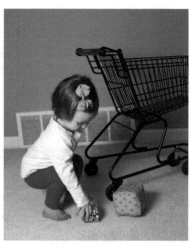

Shop 'til you drop

You can also encourage squatting by having your child push a toy shopping cart and pick up toys you've placed along the floor. She can walk along and squat to pick them up. Plus having the shopping cart available gives your child extra support for her arms so she doesn't have to fully rely on her leg strength. If you don't have a shopping cart or push toy, sit down behind your child while she is standing and facing away from you. Place an appealing toy on the floor in front of her. As she begins to squat, hold her at her hips, providing some support. Then, as she gains control while reaching for the toy, slowly decrease your amount of assistance.

Activity #4: Mr Tambourine Man

This activity requires making 2 homemade tambourines.

Once the tambourines are complete, you and your child can play an imitation game with them. Stand facing your little one and give her a tambourine while you hold yours in one hand. Demonstrate how to shake it to make noise. Encourage your child to do the same. Once she understands how to shake it, show her how to hold it with one hand and

Homemade Toy **Toddler Tambourine**

Take 2 sturdy paper plates and tape them securely together halfway around. (Don't use Styrofoam plates; they break too easily.) Fill the tambourine half-full of dry cereal, then securely tape the paper plates together the rest of the way. Choose colorful duct tape; it's fun and works well. Repeat these steps to make the second tambourine.

tap it with the other. As your child imitates you, praise her by saying, "Good job!"

If your child seems to be having fun, continue the activity. Encourage her to copy you as you tap the tambourine against your hip, over your head, and in various directions. Both of you will have a blast making music together. Plus, this activity is great for your little one's motor skills.

Activity #5: Chugga, Chugga, Choo Choo!

After your child is walking independently, she may still enjoy participating in activities that encourage crawling. Crawling while pushing and pulling a toy, such as a homemade choo-choo train, is a fun option.

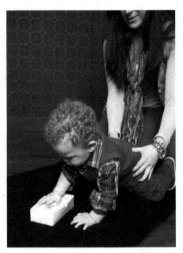

What child doesn't love a choo-choo train? You can bet that your little one will get a kick out of a simple homemade train.

Show her how to load and unload items and how to pull the train around. You may want to get creative and make a short tunnel for her to push the train

Chugga, chugga, choo choo!

through. This provides an ideal opportunity to talk about the concepts of through and under.

Homemade Toy Choo-choo Train

Take several small boxes (milk cartons or individual-sized cereal boxes will work) and tie them together with short pieces of ribbon. They should slide easily so that your child can pull the train. If they don't slide nicely, stick several squares of contact paper on the bottom of each box. Cut the tops out of several of the boxes so that your child can load them with a small toy or snack.

Activity #6: Come Fly Away

Lie on your back and bring your hips
and knees toward your chin, making a level platform out of your shins.
Place your child facing you on your
shins and hold her securely around
her rib cage just under her arms.
Slightly extend and flex your hips and
knees to make your child bounce in
the air. Now sing "Come Fly Away"
as your child flies! Be sure to hold
on tight.

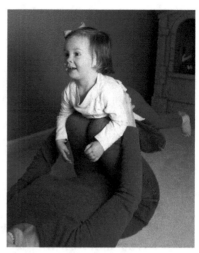

Come fly away

Activity #7: Getting to the Point

Pointing is a form of communication. With just one gesture, a child
uses her index finger to show you something she wants or to bring your
attention to something. Children can have fun with pointing games. Ask
your child questions like, "Where is your nose? Where are your eyes?
Where is Mommy?" Encourage her to answer questions by pointing;
demonstrate pointing if she doesn't point spontaneously.

When she wants something, don't automatically give it to her if she
reaches for it or grunts; give her a verbal prompt her to point at it, such
as, "Can you point to the drink and say 'drink,' please?" Never pass up a
teaching opportunity!

Activity #8: Poking Fun!

You can have your little one continue to practice her pointing skills by
having her pretend to dial numbers on a toy phone or peck on an old
keyboard. Glue different textures of fabric at the bottom of each section
of an egg carton or old ice tray and show your child how to point with
her index finger to feel and poke at the various textures. She will enjoy
the activity, and it is wonderful for practicing isolating her index finger.

Activity #9: Go Find!

You can also play the "go find" game by pointing to a toy and saying, "Can you find the red fire truck?" Make sure that your child sees you looking at the toy as you point at it. Once she finds the toy, tell her, "Good! You found the fire truck! Now can you find the red ball?" Be sure to look at the ball and point at it. It's likely that your child will enjoy this game, and all the while she will be improving her communication skills.

Activity #10: Blow It Out

This is a good age to start teaching your child about the concept of blowing. Begin by holding a tissue in front of your mouth. Blow on the tissue so that it moves; then say, "Look, Mommy blew on the tissue and made it move." You can also demonstrate blowing out candles and blowing bubbles in milk using a straw. Give your little one an opportunity to try it out. This activity helps improve breath control, which is good for speech skills. Don't worry if your child doesn't catch on right away. It can take a while to learn the skill of blowing.

Emerging Skill: Scribbling

You may have noticed that your child finds it fascinating when you are making out a grocery list or writing a check. She may even attempt to confiscate your pen or pencil on occasion. At this age, it's appropriate to let her scribble on a piece of paper using a crayon. This teaches cause and effect, and you can also teach her colors during the activity.

At this age, your child probably holds the crayon with a fisted grasp or with her thumb and first finger toward the paper with the rest of her fingers wrapped around the crayon. This is typical for her age.

Educational and Online Videos: Avoid Exposure Prior to 18 Months of Age According to the American Academy of Pediatrics

Every parent wants to know, "Do educational videos actually help babies learn?" According to the research, probably not. One study found no difference in language acquisition between children who watched educational shows and those who didn't.[101] Other research suggests that babies learn language better by interacting with live speakers than by passively listening to language coming from a screen.[13,102] Another study found that educational television (TV) shows for toddlers can limit adult-child interactions and affect the back-and-forth conversations needed for language development.[103] Most importantly, the time that a child spends watching screens is time that could be spent learning through engaging and interacting with parents, siblings, and caregivers.[13] For example, during an interaction, Mom might say, "Look—it's a bird! The bird says, 'Tweet, tweet'! What does it say?" Her child gains new information and also has to recall that information by answering the question. When the question is answered correctly, Mom can reinforce her child's success by saying, "Good job! You're right. The bird says, 'Tweet, tweet'!" When it comes to teaching language to children younger than 2 years, social interaction beats educational videos hands down.

Smartphones and Tablets

Approximately 75% of young children have a tablet, and many start using tablets and mobile devices before their first birthday.[104,105] Some parents believe that swiping and pinching the touch screens on smartphones and tablets is good for their child's fine motor skills. However, that is not the case. Research suggests that screen time is negatively associated with fine motor and hand skills in young children.[106]

Be aware that interruptions from cell phones alter the interactions you have with you child, negatively affecting her opportunities for learning.[107] Also, the presence of a tablet can change the parent-child dynamic.[108]

Tablet and smartphone applications (apps) that target infants and preschoolers exist on the market and are often labeled as "educational." Keep in mind that there is limited research that shows babies learn skills that can be used in the real world from screens.[109] Early, excessive media exposure can be harmful to early development. The American Academy of Pediatrics recommendation is to avoid devices until your child is 18 months old, with one exception: video chatting.

Video Chat

Young children can learn language and participate in social interactions through live video chatting.[110] Many families with young children live apart from grandparents and other extended family members. Yet, these relationships are very important for adults as well as children. One way to foster connection between those at a geographic distance is through video chatting. Make the chat fun, engaging, and meaningful by reading a book or singing a song. Another fun activity is to give the child simple directions to carry out, such as, "Touch your nose!" or "Put your hands over your ears!" It is also important to ensure that the child has a clear view of the adult's face on the screen. When an adult video chats with a young child, be sure to keep it brief. Don't let the chat go on too long, and if your toddler seems to be losing attention, it's probably time to change things up or sign off.

Fun Alternatives to Screen Time

Activity #1: Coloring My World

Playing and coloring on a vertical surface puts your child's wrist in an extended position, which is the same way the wrist is held when writing and cutting. Coloring in this position also strengthens the muscles in her shoulders, which, together with her trunk muscles, form a base of support for her arms and hands. A solid base supports the many fine motor skills your child will develop in the future. She can strengthen this base by coloring or finger painting a picture while she stands. If you don't have an easel, tape an extra-large piece of paper to the wall. (Butcher paper works well.) Even though the paper is taped in place, prompt your child to stabilize it with one hand as she scribbles with the other to encourage bilateral skills.

Activity #2: Painting the Town

If your child enjoys coloring, she will probably love finger painting. Have her sit in a high chair with a tray for this activity if possible. Use the recipe for edible finger paint or a tiny bit of vanilla or chocolate pudding. Tape a large piece of thick paper to her tray (wax paper and heavy-duty

Homemade Edible Finger Paint

To create edible finger paint, you will need the following ingredients:
- Three-fourths cup corn flour
- Six tablespoons sugar
- Four-and-a-half cups water
- Natural food coloring—various colors

In a saucepan, mix corn flour and sugar together. Turn heat to medium and slowly add water. Heat until mixture thickens. Cool slightly and split into 4 equal portions. Add food coloring as desired. It will thicken as it cools.

This homemade finger paint keeps for as long as a week in airtight containers.

foil are also options) and give her a small bowl of paint or pudding. Show her how to use her index finger to make circles and other designs on the paper. She may even imitate you as you draw vertical or horizontal lines. If she doesn't, try placing your hand over hers, guiding her through several strokes. As you draw the stroke, tell her what you're doing by saying, "We're making a line that goes down," or "We're making a circle." Remove your hand and demonstrate the stroke again while repeating what you said. See if your child imitates the stroke. If so, repeat the verbal cue by saying, "Great, you are making a line that goes down."

At this age, if your child has no interest in imitating strokes, don't worry about it. Let her enjoy working on her own artistic creation. The point is for her to have tons of fun!

Activity #3: Call Me

Have you ever noticed your child watching you as you talk on the phone? She is learning constantly, especially while watching you. If you give her your phone, she'll probably put it straight to her ear. She may even already have her own toy phone. Either way, have some fun playing this phone game with her.

Sit your child on your lap, hold a phone to your ear, and speak into it, mentioning your child's name. "I'm having fun with Susie today. She's right here with me. Would you like her to say hello?" Hold the phone to your child's ear and say, "Susie, say hello to the person on the phone." Continue a conversation using words your child is familiar with, such as mommy and daddy. Occasionally put the phone to your child's ear to see if she will talk into it.

Homemade Toy *Beanbag Toss*

To make a homemade beanbag game, find
- Two pairs of colorful, old socks (Make sure they don't have holes in them.)
- A large bag of dried beans
- A large cardboard box

Fill the socks with beans, leaving room for the beans to jiggle around. Securely stitch the sock closed so it's roughly the size of your fist when complete. For textured beanbags that provide sensory input, stitch together 4-inch squares of various textured fabrics to make the bags. There are all sorts of possibilities—corduroy, velveteen, fake fur, wool, even leather. Your child will love these "feely" beanbags.

Cut out a large hole in the center of the box and 2 smaller holes on either side of the center hole. The beanbags should fit easily through the holes. It's fun to decorate the box so you have 3 faces. The beanbag holes become the mouths for each face.

Time to play! To play the game, show your child how to toss a beanbag into one of the holes. It's fine if she stands directly above the box and drops them in. Go crazy with excitement every time she gets one through the target. "Way to go! What a good job! You hit the target! You threw it through the hole!" Once all 4 bags have made it through the targets, have your child help you open the box and remove them for another round of the game. As your child gets older, have her back away from the box to make the task more challenging. You can also eventually teach her different ways to toss beanbags, such as underhand and overhand.

Activity #4: Here's the Scoop

A super easy and fun activity involves scooping and pouring. Select a small storage bin with a lid and add a box of dry cereal. Use small cups that your child can grasp easily and show her how to scoop a bit of cereal using a cup. Demonstrate how much fun she can have pouring from one cup to another. Add a baby spoon to the mix and show her how to scoop cereal with the spoon, putting it into the cups. This is wonderful practice for self-feeding!

Activity #5: Pulling Ahead

When your child is standing up, show her how to use a pull toy. Have her hold the string of the pull toy and encourage her to take several steps and pull the toy along behind her. Have her follow you around corners and difference pieces of furniture in the room, or take her outside and see if she can pull it over uneven surfaces such as the driveway or lawn. Be sure that the string on the pull toy is short so it doesn't pose a strangulation risk. Supervise your child closely while using the toy and put it away in a safe place when playtime is over.[111]

Activity #6: Mix and Match

Your toddler is gaining all kinds of new skills, such as noticing how items are similar and different. That means this is the perfect time to play a matching game. Teach her how to match similar objects, such as cups, dolls, socks, spoons, and articles of clothing. It's also fun to take photographs of familiar people, household pets, and favorite objects; have duplicate copies made; and laminate or cover them with contact paper. Place them out on a table and show your child how to pair them together. Now it's her turn! Keep them in a shoebox so that you can pull this activity out on a rainy day.

Activity #7: The Long and Winding Road

Learning to walk is a challenging feat, so it's important to make sure your child has plenty of opportunities to practice this skill. Show her how to walk while pushing a large box or rolling chair. This is a nice exercise for strength and balance.

Another super-fun activity that is great for balance, coordination, and motor planning skills is for your child to navigate an obstacle course. You can create the course based on your child's ability level. First, scan the room and remove all unsafe objects that pose a danger to your child, such as sharp edges and breakable items. Take large boxes, cushions, pillows, chairs, laundry baskets, and anything else that you can find and arrange them into a fun obstacle course for your little one to navigate through. There should be opportunities for a variety of skills, including climbing over, crawling under, and walking around. A table with a blanket over it makes an excellent tunnel. If possible, go through the course first and have your toddler follow you. Add language to the activity by telling your child, "What fun! You are climbing over a pillow and going through a tunnel!" You can add some music to the activity for extra fun.

Activity #8: I Get Around

As soon as your child starts taking steps, providing a push toy will give her the opportunity to practice her walking and balance skills. Children love toy grocery carts! At first, kneel behind your child and hold her at the hips as she takes steps, at least until she becomes more stable with walking.

If you don't have a push toy, you can use a child-sized chair or large box. To help the chair slide across the

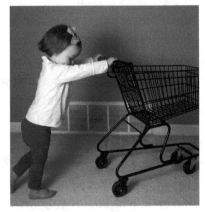

I get around

floor, you can cut slits in 4 tennis balls and place them on the chair feet.

If your child still has difficulty pushing the chair or box forward, give her a little help, but take it slowly.

Activity #9: Do You Hear What I Hear?

This is a fun activity that will help your child discover a variety of sounds. Record different noises, such as the garbage truck, fire engines, a family member's voice, a toilet flushing, or a dog barking. Play each sound back and ask your child to identify it. You might play the dog barking and ask her, "Is that a dog or a cat?" If she says dog, say, "Yes! That was the dog saying, 'Bark, bark'!" It's a good idea to include sounds like fire engines and a toilet flushing so that your child won't be frightened when she hears them.

Activity #10: Stomp Your Stuff

For this activity, you will need a sturdy squeaky toy. Place it in front of your child and show her how to stomp it with her foot to make it squeak. Practice counting by having her stomp 1, 2, and 3 times!

Emerging Skill: Stacking 4 to 6 Blocks

Even though stacking blocks is a challenging skill, children are always intrigued by this activity! Not only does it require the skill of grasping and manipulating the blocks, but motor planning skills are necessary to position the blocks properly. During this age range, these skills are improving and your child is developing more control as she grasps and releases items, which makes block stacking easier. It's important to provide a variety of stacking toys such as blocks and rings at this age; your child will enjoy experimenting with these.

Television and Other Screens: Avoid Use Up to 18 Months of Age Except for Video Chatting, According to the American Academy of Pediatrics

Letting your child watch a 30-minute TV show may seem like the perfect opportunity to get some housework done or start dinner, but there are other alternatives you may want to try first. Why?

Studies suggest that most children don't understand what they see on a screen at this early age, which means they can't learn anything from shows that claim to be educational.[112] Lights, sudden scene changes, and various sounds may be overstimulating to a young, developing brain.[15] A recent study revealed that children exposed to more than 2 hours of screen time a day had a 7.7-fold risk of being diagnosed with attention-deficit/hyperactivity disorder.[113]

It's also a good idea to limit the amount of background TV your child is exposed to. Research suggests that background TV distracts a baby,[114,115] affecting her ability to play, and play is important for babies because it's how they learn about the world. Unfortunately, research reveals that 39% of families with a baby or young child report almost always having a TV on as background noise.[116] Television causes parents to interact less with their children, resulting in less bonding and exposure to language.

So if the TV is out of the picture, what's a busy parent to do? One option that my children enjoyed are audiobooks. I absolutely love the public library; I am a regular there, checking out audiobooks. Take advantage of these and you'll find your little one engaged and entertained while being exposed to an abundance of language and interesting stories. If you or a sibling aren't available to hold up the book and turn the pages, just turn the audio on and let your child be entertained listening to the story! But remember, reading a book to a child is a significantly different experience than hearing it. Making up magical stories to tell your child helps to create her imagination.

A super-fun alternative to TV is to record your voice reading several of your child's favorite stories. Use fun, animated voices and change your pitch for the voices of different characters. Ask your child an

 Tip   *When You Can Watch Your Shows*

To limit background television exposure, record your favorite shows and watch them only when your child is not in the room or, better yet, while she's sleeping.

occasional question after you have read the text like, "Do you like kitty cats? Does the kitty cat say, 'Meow'?" This is the perfect treat for your little one to enjoy while you perform a pressing household duty.

Another option? Music! Children love music. Figure out some of her favorite tunes and make your child her very own soundtrack. Be sure to play the soundtrack only when you have important tasks to complete. That way, listening to these songs will be a special treat for you and your child!

Activities That Trump Screens

Activity #1: Stack It Up

When you are teaching your child to stack blocks, it's a good idea to start with large blocks and progress to smaller ones. You can begin with empty boxes from the pantry and progress to smaller boxes, and you also have your set of upcycled blocks. Once your little one is ready to stack tabletop blocks, begin with 2 to 3 blocks. Demonstrate by placing one on top of the other. Give her an opportunity to stack the blocks. If she doesn't seem to understand, place one block on the table and one in her hand and tap the block on the table. "Put your block on top of this block." If she attempts the task several times and is unable to position one on top of the other, add sticky Velcro on the blocks to help her out at first.

You can also have her stack the blocks against a wall or in the corner of a box to help with alignment. Once she understands the importance of lining up the blocks, you can back away from the wall or corner and remove the Velcro. This is a great activity because it requires eye-hand coordination, fine motor skills, and visual skills. Always encourage your child to knock the tower over once she's finished. That will bring a smile to her face!

Truth Be Told

At close to 24 months of age, your child may begin to show a preference toward her right or left hand. However, many children don't demonstrate a tendency toward handedness for another year or two. Don't try to force your toddler to use any particular hand; rather, let her make the selection that feels most natural for her.

Activity #2: *Tie a Yellow Ribbon*

Select 2 containers, one with an opening that your child's hand will fit inside and one with a narrow opening, such as a honey bottle. Decorate them with nontoxic paint pens if you wish. You'll need ribbons of different colors, widths, and textures, none more than 6 inches long. Put all of the ribbons inside the container with the larger opening. Show your child how to take a ribbon out of one container. Then have her use her index finger to push each ribbon into the opening of the honey container. This is another activity that is quite simple but extremely entertaining and wonderful for fine motor skills! When she wants to have another go at the activity, she may need some help getting the ribbons out of the smaller container.

Activity #3: *The Muffin Man*

Have some fine motor fun with pom-pom play. For this activity you will need a muffin tin or ice tray out of your kitchen, an empty wet-wipe container, and a bag of colorful pom-poms (found at a craft or dollar store). Your child will enjoy putting the pom-poms in the individual muffin holes and removing them. Have her transfer the pom-poms from one container to the other. You can also teach your child how to match and sort the pom-poms by color. This is a fun and fantastic way to work on pincer grasp and eye-hand coordination. Never leave your child's side during this activity to ensure that a pom-pom doesn't end up in her mouth.

Activity #4: *Wipeout*

Using the homemade wipeout toy, encourage your child to use her index finger to press the button to open the wet-wipe container. Once the top pops open, make sure that a bit of the fabric square is showing. If your child doesn't reach for the fabric to pull it out of the container, demonstrate how to pinch it with your thumb and index finger. Encourage her to pinch the fabric with one hand while holding the wipe container with the opposite hand. She may need a little assistance securing the container against her body with her arm. Prompt her to pull the fabric pieces out of the container. This is great for using 2 hands together, grasping, and pinching.

Homemade Wipeout Toy [117]

Have you ever given your child a wet-wipe container to keep her occupied? It's an absolute treat to pull the wipes out of the container and scatter them all over the floor. Here is a fun idea shared by Kim at ASpottedPony.com for upcycling a wipe container into a toy that your child will play with over and over. Get ready for hours of stimulating and productive play for your toddler!

There is so much about this toy that you will love! It is quiet, cute, safe, stimulating, inexpensive, and repurposing things you already have. Tiny fingers love to push the little button to open the door and pull out the little pieces of colorful fabric.

The first step is to use up the wipes in a container (that's easy enough with a little one in the house). Then collect pieces of fabric from around the house. This can be as easy or elaborate as you would like. Use scrap fabric pieces and applique numbers, letters, and shapes onto the fabric if you are ambitious. While playing with your child you can work on number, letter, and shape recognition. Different textures, patterns, and colors are also great for making her excited to see and feel what is coming next.

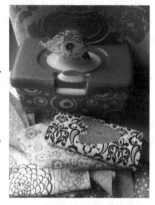

Wipeout toy

If you don't have fabric lying around, just cut up pieces of old T-shirts or towels. Hem all the edges or just leave them raw; it's up to you. Cut the pieces to about the size of a DVD case. Usually about 20 squares is the perfect amount to fit in the container.

This would be a special gift to make and give to expecting moms or for a first birthday!

Activity #5: A Balancing Act

Once your child walks independently, she is familiar with shifting her weight from one side to the other. She may be able to stand on one foot alone or with some help from you. While she is standing, show her how you can stand on one foot. Stand in front of her, take her hands, then lift your foot and ask her to do the same. If she doesn't imitate you, rock from foot to foot while singing a song and see if she'll join in. As she gains strength and confidence, it won't be long before she's able to stand on one foot for several seconds. This is an important skill because it is a precursor to putting on a pair of pants or shorts.

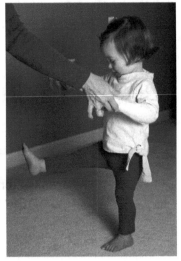

A balancing act

Activity #6: Jump for Joy

If you have a firm sofa or chair cushion, place it on the floor. Have your toddler stand in the middle of the cushion. Bend your knees and say, "Look, I'm bending my knees. Can you bend your knees like Mommy?" Then demonstrate a big jump. Take both of your child's hands and repeat your knee-bending demonstration. "Look, I'm bending my knees. Can you bend your knees like me?" After your child bends her knees, tell her to jump, and as her feet come off the cushion, give her some assistance by gently guiding her up into the jump as you are holding her hands. Praise her for her success by saying, "Good job! What a wonderful jumper you are!"

Activity #7: Eggs-actly Right!

Have you ever wondered what to do with leftover plastic eggs? Here is a wonderful activity that gives you something to do with those eggs and helps your child work on her grasping and bilateral skills. All you need are 6 or 8 plastic eggs and 3 or 4 colorful old socks. Cut the toe out of a sock and demonstrate how to put an egg inside the sock. You can reach into the other end of the sock and pull the egg through, or you can use 2 hands and squeeze the sock to work the egg to the other end of the sock. Give your child a chance to try the task and encourage her to push the egg in both directions. Although it sounds like a simple task, your child will be thoroughly entertained. It's likely she will want to repeat the activity again and again. If the eggs tend to come apart, just glue the sides together with nontoxic glue prior to the activity.

Activity #8: Let the Good Times Roll

As your toddler gets close to age 2, she will likely show an interest in kicking a ball. If she doesn't attempt this on her own, you can teach her this skill. If you are indoors, let your toddler go barefoot so she can feel the ball touch her toes. Start by demonstrating how to kick a large, light-weight ball, such as a blow-up beach ball. Once your child is able to kick a stationary ball, you can try rolling the ball toward her. When the ball nears her foot, say, "Kick the ball!" If the ball even touches her foot, praise her by saying, "Good job! You kicked the ball!" With a little practice, she'll master this skill in no time.

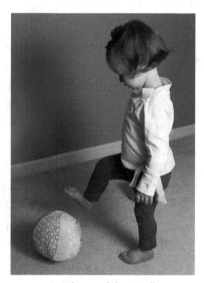

Let the good times roll

Activity #9: Sock It to Me!

Did you know that children typically learn to remove clothing before they learn to put it on? This activity will help your child learn to remove her socks. Just place a loose sock on your child's foot and encourage her to take it off. You might need to demonstrate first or provide hand-over-hand assistance. Another way to teach the concept of taking off is to slip a loose scrunchy (a fabric-covered elastic band used for fastening the hair) over her toes or foot and ask her to remove it. The scrunchy is easy to grasp, and she likely won't need as much assistance to remove it.

Activity #10: Copycat

Ask your little one to imitate your body movements. For example, cover your mouth with your hand and ask her to do the same. Start with simple positions and gradually progress to those that are more challenging. For example, hold one hand over your head and put one hand on your belly and ask her to copy you. Another fun position for her to copy is hands on hips. You may need to give her some guidance at first, but she'll eventually catch on.

What a Year!

Your baby has grown into a busy toddler who loves exploring her world. The phrase "never a dull moment" has likely taken on a whole new meaning now that your little one is constantly on the go. As your child continues to explore her world and gain new skills, her confidence will grow. With her expanding vocabulary and ability to use gestures, you will find it easier to communicate with your little one.

By spending quality time with your child and carrying out the activities in this book, you have played a significant role in her development and solidified the bond between you two. Your little one has a big future ahead; thanks to you, she has a solid foundation for further development. Continue to play with your toddler and carry out fun, developmentally stimulating activities. You'll find there is nothing better than rediscovering the world right along with your child.

American Academy of Pediatrics Media Use Guidelines[118]

- Discourage use of screen media for babies younger than 18 months other than video chatting.
- For children 18 to 24 months, parents may select high-quality educational programming and watch the content with their toddler to help the child understand what is on the screen.
- Children between ages 2 and 5 years should limit media use to less than 1 hour per day of high-quality shows, and parents should watch with them to explain the media content and apply it to real life.
- Do not expose children to fast-paced, distracting, or violent content.

- Screens and devices should be powered off when not in use.
- Parents should designate "media-free" periods, such as mealtime and bedtime.
- No screens in the hour before bedtime, and no devices in the bedroom when sleeping.
- Children 6 years and older should have consistent limits set for media use, and parents should ensure that the media does not interfere with sleep, physical exercise, and other healthy activities.

Epilogue

You now have the knowledge and tools to make play an enjoyable and stimulating part of your baby's daily routine. Keep it simple, be flexible, and incorporate what works for you and your baby. When time allows throughout the day, do your best to use the age-appropriate activities introduced in this book.

It's important to find balance between supportive play and overstimulation. Always start slowly and remain relaxed to encourage your baby to relax as well. Be sensitive to your baby's needs and communication. Remember, when your little one disengages by turning or looking away, this is a sign that your baby needs a break.

Do your best to limit your baby's time in baby gear and avoid exposure to television, videos, and other technology. The following chart includes specific guidelines for the use of the various baby products that were included in this book. Use this quick guide anytime you need to refresh your memory about a specific product, and always follow product manufacturers' guidelines for the safe use of products. Whenever possible, limit your baby's total time in various pieces of equipment to between 2 and 3 hours each day (less is better). Don't forget to frequently reposition your baby and provide plenty of tummy time and side lying during play.

In the early days and months after your baby's birth, it's easy to become overwhelmed with the responsibilities of parenting. Slow down, take a deep breath, and remember to take care of yourself. Get plenty of rest, eat well, and try to balance the demands of everyday life and being a new parent by setting aside some time for you. You can only be the best for your baby if you are mentally and physically where you need to be. Don't be afraid to ask for help when you need it. Your friends and family are there to support you.

Product	Comments	Maximum Time Recommended for Use
Bath seat	Avoid use—unsafe.	None
Bouncer seat	Follow recommendations in Chapter 7.	30 minutes a day
Bumbo baby seat	Always supervise your baby during use.	15 minutes a day
Bumper pad	Avoid use—unsafe.	None
Car safety seat	Use only when riding in a motor vehicle.	Varies
Carrier	Use when necessary, but remember to hold and carry your baby whenever possible.	Varies
Changing table with fewer than 4 sides	Avoid use—unsafe.	None
Co-sleeper/bedside sleeper	Avoid use—unsafe.	None
Drop-side crib	Avoid use—unsafe.	None
Educational video	Avoid use up to age 2 years.	None
Jumping device	Avoid use—unsafe.	None
Portable rocking sleeper	Follow recommendations in Chapter 6.	30 minutes a day
Sleep positioner	Avoid use—unsafe.	None
Smart toy	Follow recommendations in Chapter 9.	Limit use.
Stationary activity center	Follow recommendations in Chapter 8.	15 minutes a day
Swing	Follow recommendations in Chapter 7.	30 minutes a day
Television	Avoid use up to age 2 years.	None
Walker	Avoid use—unsafe.	None
Walking harness	Follow recommendations in Chapter 9.	5 to 10 minutes at a time

As parents, we want our children to be the best and brightest. We want to make it possible for them to go to the best preschools so they can get into the finest schools and attend challenging universities.

From the first days of our children's lives, we try to do everything just right for them, yet sometimes our best intentions fall short. As Maya Angelou says, "When you know better you do better."

Now that it's known how the overuse of baby gear, educational videos, television, and smart toys has the potential to negatively affect our children's development, let's do something about it. Let's do our best to cut back on the use of baby gear and eliminate screen time in the first 2 years of our children's lives.

As a society, parents, caregivers, pediatricians, and other professionals need to come together and acknowledge that something needs to change. We absolutely cannot afford to put the future of our children in jeopardy. Therefore, we must commit to limiting their time with these devices and spend more time touching, hugging, playing with, and communicating with our little ones.

I sincerely hope this book has provided the information you need to understand the crucial role you can play in your baby's development. You can help your little one thrive by spending time together, bonding, playing, and supporting your baby's learning. This precious time with your little one passes quickly, so take advantage of every moment!

References

1. US Department of Agriculture. 2015 expenditures on children by families. Accessed October 27, 2021. https://www.fns.usda.gov/resource/2015-expenditures-children-families

2. Kotulak R. *Inside the Brain: Revolutionary Discoveries of How the Mind Works.* Andrews and McMeel; 1997

3. Schiller P. Early brain development research review and update. *Brain Development Exchange.* November/December 2010:26–30

4. Littlefield TR, Kelly KM, Reiff JL, Pomatto JK. Car seats, infant carriers, and swings: their role in deformational plagiocephaly. *J Prosthet Orthot.* 2003;15(3):102–106

5. Branch LG, Kesty K, Krebs E, Wright L, Leger S, David LR. Deformational plagiocephaly and craniosynostosis: trends in diagnosis and treatment after the "back to sleep" campaign. *J Craniofac Surg.* 2015;26(1):147–150

6. Pin T, Eldridge B, Galea MP. A review of the effects of sleep position, play position and equipment use on motor development of infants. *Dev Med Child Neurol.* 2007;49(11):858–867

7. Christakis DA, Gilkerson J, Richards JA, et al. Audible television and decreased adult words, infant vocalizations, and conversational turns: a population based study. *Arch Pediatr Adolesc Med.* 2009;163(6):554–558

8. Zimmerman FJ, Christakis DA. Children's television viewing and cognitive outcomes: a longitudinal analysis of national data. *Arch Pediatr Adolesc Med.* 2005;159(7):619–625

9. Christakis DA, Zimmerman FJ, DiGiuseppe DL, McCarty CA. Early television exposure and subsequent attentional problems in children. *Pediatrics.* 2004;113(4):708–713

10. Hancox RJ, Poulton R. Watching television is associated with childhood obesity: but is it clinically important? *Int J Obes (Lond).* 2006;30(1):171–175

11. Manganello JA, Taylor CA. Television exposure as a risk factor for aggressive behavior among 3-year-old children. *Arch Pediatr Adolesc Med.* 2009;163(11):1037–1045

12. Thompson DA, Christakis DA. The association between television viewing and irregular sleep schedules among children less than 3 years of age. *Pediatrics.* 2005;116(4):851–856

13. American Academy of Pediatrics. AAP announces new recommendations for children's media use. HealthyChildren.org. Published October 21, 2016. Accessed October 27, 2021. https://www.healthychildren.org/English/news/Pages/AAP-Announces-New-Recommendations-for-Childrens-Media-Use.aspx

14. Bleses D, Makransky G, Dale PS, Højen A, Ari BA. Early productive vocabulary predicts academic achievement 10 years later. *Appl Psycholinguist.* 2016;37:1461–1476

15. Christakis DA. The effects of fast-paced cartoons. *Pediatrics.* 2011;128(4):772–774

16. Rideout V, Hammel E. *The Media Family: Electronic Media in the Lives of Infants, Toddlers, Preschoolers and their Parents.* Kaiser Family Foundation; 2006

17. Troseth GL, DeLoache JS. The medium can obscure the message: young children's understanding of video. *Child Dev.* 1998;69(4):950–965

18. Schmitt KL, Anderson DR. Television & reality: toddlers' use of visual information from video to guide behavior. *Media Psychol.* 2002;4(1):51–76

19. American Academy of Pediatrics. HealthyChildren.org. Accessed October 27, 2021. http://www.healthychildren.org

20. Bly L. *Motor Skill Acquisition in the First Year: An Illustrated Guide to Normal Development.* Therapy Skill Builders; 1994

21. Consumer Reports. Should you buy a baby walker? Published July 3, 2007. Accessed October 27, 2021. https://www.consumerreports.org/cro/news/2007/07/should-you-buy-a-baby-walker/index.htm

22. Gardner HG; American Academy of Pediatrics Committee on Injury, Violence, and Poison Prevention. Office-based counseling for unintentional injury prevention. *Pediatrics.* 2007;119(1):202–206

23. American Academy of Pediatrics Task Force on Infant Sleep Positioning and SIDS. Positioning and SIDS. *Pediatrics.* 1992;89(6):1120–1126

24. Davis BE, Moon RY, Sachs HC, Ottolini MC. Effects of sleep position on infant motor development. *Pediatrics.* 1998;102(5):1135–1140

25. World Health Organization Multicenter Growth Reference Study Group. WHO Motor Development Study: windows of achievement for six gross motor development milestones. *Acta Paediatr Suppl.* 2006;450:86–95

26. Hattangadi N, Cost KT, Birken CS, et al. Parenting stress during infancy is a risk factor for mental health problems in 3-year-old children. *BMC Public Health.* 2020;20(1):1726

27. Kranowitz CS. *The Out of Sync Child: Recognizing and Coping with Sensory Processing Disorder.* Perigee Book; 2005

28. American Academy of Pediatrics. Infant vision development: what can babies see? HealthyChildren.org. Updated January 5, 2012. Accessed October 27, 2021. https://www.healthychildren.org/English/ages-stages/baby/Pages/Babys-Vision-Development.aspx

29. American Optometric Association. Infant vision: birth to 24 months of age. Accessed October 27, 2021. https://www.aoa.org/healthy-eyes/eye-health-for-life/infant-vision?sso=y

30. Saffran JR, Werker JF, Werner LA. The infant's auditory world: hearing, speech, and the beginnings of language. In: Kuhn D, Siegler RS, eds. *Handbook of Child Psychology: Vol. 2: Cognition, Perception, and Language.* 6th ed. John Wiley & Sons; 2006:58–108

31. Chiocca EM. *Advanced Pediatric Assessment.* Lippincott Williams & Wilkins; 2011

32. Mennella JA, Beauchamp GK. Infants' exploration of scented toys: effects of prior experiences. *Chem Senses.* 1998;23(1):11–17

33. Ayres AJ, Robbins J. *Sensory Integration and the Child: Understanding Hidden Sensory Challenges.* 25th anniversary ed. Western Psychological Services; 2005

34. Goldberg JM, Wilson VJ, Cullen KE, et al. *The Vestibular Sense: A Sixth Sense.* Oxford University Press; 2012

35. Bundy AC, Lane S, Murray EA, Fisher AG. *Sensory Integration: Theory and Practice.* 2nd ed. F.A. Davis; 2002

36. Cameron OG. *Visceral Sensory Neuroscience: Interoception.* Oxford University Press; 2002

37. American Academy of Pediatrics Section on Complementary and Integrative Medicine and Council on Children with Disabilities. Sensory integration therapies for children with developmental and behavioral disorders. *Pediatrics.* 2012;129(6):1186–1189

38. Sensory Processing Disorder Foundation. Sensory processing disorder checklist. Accessed October 27, 2021. http://www.spdfoundation.net/library/checklist.html

39. American Academy of Pediatrics Task Force on Sudden Infant Death Syndrome. The changing concept of sudden infant death syndrome: diagnostic coding shifts, controversies regarding the sleeping environment, and new variables to consider in reducing risk. *Pediatrics.* 2005;116(5):1245–1255

40. Centers for Disease Control and Prevention. Sudden unexpected infant death and sudden infant death syndrome. Data and statistics. Reviewed April 28, 2021. Accessed October 27, 2021. https://www.cdc.gov/sids/data.htm

41. Centers for Disease Control and Prevention. Sudden unexpected infant death and sudden infant death syndrome. Reviewed December 31, 2020. Accessed October 27, 2021. http://www.cdc.gov/sids

42. American Academy of Pediatrics Task Force on Sudden Infant Death Syndrome. SIDS and other sleep-related infant deaths: updated 2016 recommendations for a safe infant sleeping environment. *Pediatrics.* 2016;138(5):e20162938

43. US Consumer Product Safety Commission. Safe sleep—cribs and infant products. Accessed October 27, 2021. https://www.cpsc.gov/SafeSleep

44. Pathways Awareness. National survey of pediatric experts indicates increase in infant delays; more tummy time is key. Accessed October 27, 2021. https://pathways.org/wp-content/uploads/2014/09/ttposterhandoutversion.pdf

45. Mildred J. Beard K, Dallwitz A, Unwin J. Play position is influenced by knowledge of SIDS sleep position recommendations. *J Pediatr Child Health.* 1995;31(6):499–502

46. Dudek-Shriber L, Zelazny S. The effects of prone positioning on the quality and acquisition of developmental milestones in four-month-old infants. *Pediatr Phys Ther.* 2007;19(1):48–55

47. Zachry AH, Nolan VG, Hand SB, Klemm SA. Infant positioning, baby gear use, and cranial asymmetry. *Matern Child Health J.* 2017;21(12):2229–2236

48. Jennings JT, Sarbaugh BG, Payne NS. Conveying the message about optimal infant positions. *Phys Occup Ther Pediatr.* 2005;25(3):3–18

49. American Academy of Pediatrics. Back to sleep, tummy to play. HealthyChildren.org. Updated January 20, 2017. Accessed October 27, 2021. https://www.healthychildren.org/English/ages-stages/baby/sleep/Pages/Back-to-Sleep-Tummy-to-Play.aspx

50. Zachry AH, Kitzmann KM. Caregiver awareness of prone play recommendations. *Am J Occup Ther.* 2011;65(1):101–105

51. Consumer Reports. Crib buying guide. Updated May 2, 2016. Accessed October 27, 2021. http://www.consumerreports.org/cro/cribs/buying-guide.htm

52. Small R. *Building Babies Better.* Trafford On Demand Publishing; 2012

53. Abbott AL, Bartlett DJ. Infant motor development and equipment use in the home. *Child Care Health Dev.* 2001;27(3):295–306

54. Littlefield TR, Beals SP, Manwaring KH, et al. Treatment of craniofacial asymmetry with dynamic orthotic cranioplasty. *J Craniofac Surg.* 1998;9(1):11–19

55. Graham JM, Kreutzman J, Earl D, Halberg A, Samayoa C, Guo X. Deformational brachycephaly in supine-sleeping infants. *J Pediatr.* 2005;146(2):253–257

56. Boere-Boonekamp MM, van der Linden–Kuiper AT. Positional preference: prevalence in infants and follow-up after two years. *Pediatrics.* 2001;107(2):339–343

57. Aarnivala H, Vuollo V, Harila V, et al. The course of positional cranial deformation from 3 to 12 months of age and associated risk factors: a follow-up with 3D imaging. *Eur J Pediatr.* 2016;175(12):1893–1903

58. Collett BR, Kartin D, Wallace ER, Cunningham ML, Speltz ML. Motor function in school-aged children with positional plagiocephaly or brachycephaly. *Pediatr Phys Ther.* 2020;32(2):107–112

59. Cheng JC, Au AW. Infantile torticollis: a review of 624 cases. *J Pediatr Orthop.* 1994;14(6):802–808

60. Luther BL. Congenital muscular torticollis. *Orthop Nurs.* 2002;21(3):21–29

61. Emery C. The determinants of treatment duration for congenital muscular torticollis. *Pediatrics.* 1994;74(10):921–929

62. Anisfeld E, Casper V, Nozyce M, Cunningham N. Does infant carrying promote attachment? An experimental study of the effects of increased physical contact on the development of attachment. *Child Dev.* 1990;61(5):1617–1627

63. Budreau G. The perceived attractiveness of preterm infants with cranial molding. *J Obstet Gynecol Neonatal Nurs.* 1989;18(1):38–44

64. Biggs WS. Diagnosis and management of positional head deformity. *Am Fam Physician.* 2003;67(9):1953–1960

65. US Food and Drug Administration. Recommendations for parents/caregivers about the use of baby products. Reviewed August 22, 2018. Accessed October 27, 2021. https://www.fda.gov/medical-devices/baby-products-sids-prevention-claims/recommendations-parents-caregivers-about-use-baby-products

66. Fish D, Lima D. An overview of positional plagiocephaly and cranial remolding orthoses. *J Prosthet Orthot.* 2003;15(2):37–45

67. St. Jude Children's Research Hospital. Do you know…torticollis (left side). Accessed October 27, 2021. https://www.stjude.org/treatment/patient-resources/caregiver-resources/patient-family-education-sheets/rehabilitation/torticollis-left-side.html

68. Anderson RC, Fielding LG, Wilson PT. Growth in reading and how children spend their time outside of school. *Read Res Q.* 1988;23(3):285–303

69. Bryant PE, Bradley L, Maclean M, Crossland J. Nursery rhymes, phonological skills and reading. *J Child Lang.* 1989;16(2):407–428

70. Dunst CJ, Meter D, Hamby DW. Relationship between young children's nursery rhyme experiences and knowledge and phonological and print-related abilities. *CELL Reviews.* 2011;4(1):1–12

71. Vittner D, McGrath J, Robinson J, et al. Increase in oxytocin from skin-to-skin contact enhances development of parent-infant relationship. *Biol Res Nurs.* 2018; 20(1):54–62

72. Mindell JA, Telofski LS, Wiegand B, Kurtz ES. A nightly bedtime routine: impact on sleep in young children and maternal mood. *Sleep.* 2009;32(5):599–606

73. Hernandez-Reif M, Diego M, Field T. Preterm infants show reduced stress behaviors and activity after 5 days of massage therapy. *Infant Behav Dev.* 2007; 30(4):557–561

74. Field T, Hernandez-Reif M. Sleep problems in infants decrease following massage therapy. *Early Child Dev Care.* 2001;168(1):95–104

75. Williams LR, Turner PR. Experiences with "babywearing": trendy parenting gear or a developmentally attuned parenting tool? *Children and Youth Services Review.* 2020;112:104918

76. Little EE, Legare CH, Carver LJ. Culture, carrying, and communication: beliefs and behavior associated with babywearing. *Infant Behav Dev.* 2019;57:101320

77. American Academy of Pediatrics. Choosing a crib. HealthyChildren.org. Updated June 10, 2021. Accessed October 27, 2021. https://www.healthychildren.org/English/ages-stages/prenatal/decisions-to-make/Pages/Choosing-a-Crib.aspx

78. Needham A, Barrett T, Peterman K. A pick-me-up for infants' exploratory skills: early simulated experiences reaching for objects using 'sticky mittens' enhances young infants' object exploration skills. *Infant Behav Dev.* 2002;25(3):279–295

79. Franchak JM. Changing opportunities for learning in everyday life: infant body position over the first year. *Infancy,* 2019;24(2):187–209

80. Ainsworth MD. Object relations, dependency and attachment: a theoretical review of the infant-mother relationship. *Child Dev.* 1969;40(4):969–1025

81. Schore AN. Effects of secure attachment relationship on right brain development, affect regulation, and infant mental health. *Infant Ment Health J.* 2001;22(1-2):7–66

82. Bertenthal BI, Van Hofsten C. Eye, head and trunk control: the foundation for manual development. *Neurosci Biobehav Rev.* 1998;22(4):515–520

83. ChildCare.gov. Selecting a child care program: visiting and asking questions. Accessed October 27, 2021. https://childcare.gov/index.php/consumer-education/selecting-a-child-care-program-visiting-and-asking-questions

84. Chess S, Thomas A. *Temperament: Theory and Practice.* Routledge; 2013

85. US Consumer Product Safety Commission. Baby seats recalled for repair by Bumbo International due to fall hazard. Published August 15, 2012. Accessed October 27, 2021. https://www.cpsc.gov/Recalls/2012/Baby-Seats-Recalled-for-Repair-by-Bumbo-International-Due-to-Fall-Hazard

86. Dix M. Why aren't babies born with bony kneecaps? Healthline. Reviewed March 27, 2019. Accessed October 27, 2021. https://www.healthline.com/health/do-babies-have-kneecaps#kneecaps-at-birth

87. Joy's Hope. Accessed October 27, 2021. http://www.joyshope.com

88. Siegel AC, Burton RV. Effects of baby walkers on motor and mental development in human infants. *J Dev Behav Pediatr.* 1999;20(5):355–361

89. American Academy of Pediatrics Committee on Injury and Poison Prevention. Injuries associated with infant walkers. *Pediatrics.* 2001;108(3):790–792

90. Deater-Deckard K, Panneton R. *Parental Stress and Early Child Development: Adaptive and Maladaptive Outcomes.* Springer; 2017

91. Bowlby J. *Attachment and Loss.* 3 vols. Basic Books; 1969–1980

92. Sosa AV. Association of the type of toy used during play with the quantity and quality of parent-infant communication. *JAMA Pediatr.* 2016;170(2):132–137

93. Wegener C, Hunt AE, Vanwanseele B, Burns J, Smith RM. Effect of children's shoes on gait: a systematic review and meta-analysis. *J Foot Ankle Res.* 2011;4:3

94. Amabile T. *The Social Psychology of Creativity.* Springer-Verlag; 1983

95. Miller BC, Gerard D. Family influences on the development of creativity in children: an integrative review. *Fam Coord.* 1979;28(3):295–312

96. Brandt A, Gebrian M, Slevc LR. Music and early language acquisition. *Front Psychol.* 2012;3:327

97. Wells G. Preschool literacy-related activities and success in school. In: Olson DR, Torrance N, Hildyard A, eds. *Literacy, Language, and Learning: The Nature and Consequences of Reading and Writing.* Cambridge University Press; 1985:229–255

98. Shore R. *Rethinking the Brain: New Insights into Early Development.* Families and Work Institute; 1997

99. Reschke PJ, Walle EA, Dukes D. Interpersonal development in infancy: the interconnectedness of emotion understanding and social cognition. *Child Dev Perspect.* 2017;11(3):178–183

100. Mindell JA, Leichman ES, DuMond C, Sadeh A. Sleep and social-emotional development in infants and toddlers. *J Clin Child Adolesc Psychol.* 2017;46(2):236–246

101. Zimmerman FJ, Christakis DA, Meltzoff AN. Associations between media viewing and language development in children under age 2 years. *J Pediatr.* 2007;151(4):364–368

102. Kirkorian HL, Choi K, Pempek TA. Toddlers' word learning from contingent and noncontingent video on touch screens. *Child Dev.* 2016;87(2):405–413

103. Christakis DA, Gilkerson J, Richards JA, et al. Audible television and decreased adult words, infant vocalizations, and conversational turns: a population-based study. *Arch Pediatr Adolesc Med.* 2009;163(6):554–558

104. Pew Research Center. Mobile fact sheet. Published April 7, 2021. Accessed October 27, 2021. https://www.pewresearch.org/internet/fact-sheet/mobile

105. Rideout V. *The Common Sense Census: Media Use by Kids Age Zero to Eight.* Common Sense Media; 2017

106. Souto PHS, Santos JN, Leite HR, et al. Tablet use in young children is associated with advanced fine motor skills. *J Mot Behav.* 2020;52(2):196–203

107. Reed J, Hirsh-Pasek K, Golinkoff RM. Learning on hold: cell phones sidetrack parent–child interactions. *Dev Psychol.* 2017;53(8):1428–1436

108. Munzer TG, Miller AL, Weeks HM, Kaciroti N, Radesky J. Differences in parent-toddler interactions with electronic versus print books. *Pediatrics.* 2019;143(4): e20182012

109. Reich SM, Yau JC, Warschauer M. Tablet-based ebooks for young children: what does the research say? *J Dev Behav Pediatr.* 2016;37(7):585–591

110. Roseberry S, Hirsh-Pasek K, Golinkoff RM. Skype me! Socially contingent interactions help toddlers learn language. *Child Dev.* 2014;85(3):956–970

111. Durbin DR; American Academy of Pediatrics Committee on Injury, Violence, and Poison Prevention. Child passenger safety. *Pediatrics.* 2011;127(4):788–793

112. Pempek TA, Kirkorian HL, Lund AF, Stevens M, Richards JE, Anderson DR. Infant responses to sequential and linguistic distortions of Teletubbies. Poster presented at: Biennial Meeting of the Society for Research in Child Development; March 27–April 1, 2007; Boston, MA

113. Tamana SK, Ezeugwu V, Chikuma J, et al. Screen-time is associated with inattention problems in preschoolers: results from the CHILD birth cohort study. *PLoS One.* 2019;14(4):e0213995

114. Kirkorian HL, Pempek TA, Murphy LA, Schmidt ME, Anderson DR. The impact of background television on parent-child interaction. *Child Dev.* 2009;80(5):1350–1359

115. Schmidt ME, Pempek TA, Kirkorian HL, Lund AF, Anderson DR. The effects of background television on the toy play behavior of very young children. *Child Dev.* 2008;79(4):1137–1151

116. Vandewater EA, Park SE, Huang X, Wartella EA. "No—you can't watch that": parental rules and young children's media use. *Am Behav Sci.* 2005;48(5):608–623

117. Bond K. Turn a wipe container into the best infant and toddler toy. A Spotted Pony. Published September 23, 2011. Accessed October 27, 2021. http://aspottedpony.com/fun-for-kids/turn-a-wipe-container-into-the-best-infant-and-toddler-toy/876

118. American Academy of Pediatrics Council on Communications and Media. Media and young minds. *Pediatrics.* 2016;138(5):e20162591

Index